ABOUT THE AUTHOR

Before studying medicine, Dr Jeff Foster completed an honours degree in Physiology at King's College London. He then went on to study medicine at Leicester–Warwick Medical School and has worked in the Midlands since qualifying in 2004. In addition to his core work as a general practitioner, until 2017 Dr Foster worked as a senior doctor in a busy accident and emergency department at Coventry Hospital.

It was through his work in general practice that Dr Foster developed an interest in men's health. After realising that this was not a dedicated speciality within medicine, he decided to create such a position in order to provide a holistic approach to the care of his male patients. Since then, Dr Foster has opened two private men's health clinics and has been involved in developing and promoting men's health at both a local and a national level. He has written medical articles on various male health topics, such as testosterone deficiency and erectile dysfunction, promoted awareness of prostate cancer and given talks to the local community.

In addition, Dr Foster writes regular articles on all aspects of health and well-being for a variety of national and international publications, including the *Sunday Mirror*, the *Guardian*, *Woman and Home* magazine, *Take a Break*, *Reader's Digest*, the *Evening Standard*, *HuffPost*, the *Daily Telegraph*, the *Daily Mail* and *Netdoctor*.

Dr Jeff Foster

MAN ALIVE

The Health Problems Men Face and How to Fix Them

PIATKUS

PIATKUS

First published in Great Britain in 2021 by Piatkus

1 3 5 7 9 10 8 6 4 2

A CIP catalogue record for this book
is available from the British Library.

ISBN: 978-0-349-42785-0

Typeset in Sabon by M Rules
Printed and bound in Great Britain by
Clays Ltd, Elcograf S.p.A

Papers used by Piatkus are from well-managed forests
and other responsible sources.

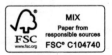

MIX
Paper from
responsible sources
FSC® C104740

Piatkus
An imprint of
Little, Brown Book Group
Carmelite House
50 Victoria Embankment
London EC4Y 0DZ

An Hachette UK Company
www.hachette.co.uk

www.littlebrown.co.uk

NOTE: the names and some details of those featured
in the case studies have been changed, or are composites,
in order to protect the privacy of individuals.

*To my wife Suzy, my son Jacob
and my daughter Gabriella*

Contents

Acknowledgements

My thanks goes to the following people:

Mr Paul Anderson for providing me with the inspiration to get involved in men's health several years ago, as well as for the hours of tutorials and advice.

Professor David Foster for always being there to offer help and guidance when I was stuck, as well as continually correcting my grammar.

Mrs Fran Foster for providing constant encouragement and allowing me to talk through ideas.

Dr Michael Foster for teaching me all I needed to know about mental health.

Mrs Susan Foster for letting me run through literally dozens of inappropriate case studies and ideas.

Dr Hilary Jones for taking the time to help me, despite no prior knowledge of who I was, and for giving me invaluable advice.

Mr Chris Lewis for providing continual urological support and advice, as well as helping me to develop my specialist interest.

Mr Ian Marber for telling me to write this book in the first place.

Mr John Watson for listening and offering advice when I needed it.

Mr Bijan Sedghi for always encouraging me to push forward and believe in my own ability.

List of Abbreviations

ADAM	Androgen Deficiency in Ageing Males questionnaire
ADHD	attention deficit hyperactivity disorder
beta-hCG	beta-human chorionic gonadotrophin
BMI	body mass index
BPH	benign prostatic hyperplasia
CBT	cognitive behavioural therapy
CVD	cardiovascular disease
DBT	dialectical behaviour therapy
DHT	dihydrotestosterone
ED	erectile dysfunction
ESWT	extracorporeal shock wave therapy
FUE	follicular unit extraction
FUT	follicular unit transplantation

HDL	high-density lipoprotein (cholesterol)
HIIT	high-intensity interval training
HRT	hormone replacement therapy (for women)
IPT	interpersonal psychotherapy
LDL	low-density lipoprotein (cholesterol)
NICE	National Institute for Health and Care Excellence
PDE5	phosphodiesterase type 5 inhibitors
PSA	prostate specific antigen test
PTSD	post-traumatic stress disorder
SHBG	sex hormone binding globulin
SSRIs	selective serotonin reuptake inhibitors
TD	testosterone deficiency
TRT	testosterone replacement therapy
TURP	transurethral resection of the prostate
WHO	World Health Organization

Why Being a Man is Bad for Your Health

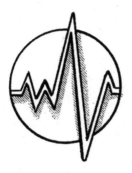

B eing a man is bad for your health. In fact, compared with women, men not only have a greater chance of contracting almost every illness but also they die sooner. And this statistic has not changed for hundreds of years. Why, then, has more effort not been put into bridging the gap between male and female health?

One problem is understanding what men's health actually is. In the media, almost every magazine and online publication dealing with men's health focuses on sex, the prostate or how to get a six-pack. But men are more than just anatomical appendages and gym routines.

When trying to define what constitutes men's health, perhaps the best place to start is looking at what makes someone a man. At six weeks of age, while in the womb, activation of the Y chromosome sets an embryo on an irreversible path towards becoming male. During puberty, the hormone testosterone's increased activity results in the majority of the features that make us appear masculine. Examples of the effects of testosterone include greater muscle mass, a deeper voice, squaring of the face and jaw, and the growth of facial hair. But testosterone alters much more than just what we can see. It changes the way we think, our mood and our personality, and it affects our kidneys, cholesterol, blood pressure and even how we produce blood. In fact, testosterone has an effect on almost every system in the body.

The idea that being a man is due solely to the influence of testosterone is, of course, simplistic, however. There are many hormonal and biochemical differences between men and women, but there are also important environmental and social factors that affect how we grow and develop into adult men. Despite initiatives to reduce gender stereotyping, being a boy still carries with it an expectation of certain behaviours and lifestyle choices; for example, boys are still commonly encouraged not to be 'soft' and not to 'cry like a girl'. In many adult couples, it is still the man who has the full-time job and his female partner who has the main childcare responsibilities. And, unlike women, it is still normal for men not to talk about their mental health with their male friends.

It is this combination of genetic, psychological and environmental factors that results in men doing so badly in matters of health; for example, in their outcomes to the main life-threatening illnesses, the differences between the two sexes are alarming. Men are more likely to die from heart disease, are at an increased risk of high blood pressure, diabetes and stroke, are more likely to get cancer and have higher rates of both trauma and suicide. Doctors have known this for decades, so why are there not more men's health specialists?

Over recent years, we have seen some badly needed improvements in the treatment of many female health problems, and we have a much better understanding of specifically female diseases and conditions, such as post-natal depression, breast cancer, cervical cancer and the negative impact menopause can have on health and well-being. Not so long ago, women suffered with high rates of post-birth complications, there was no national breast or cervical screening programme and the potentially life-altering effects of menopause were dismissed as just 'going through the change'. Now, thankfully, we have started to turn the tide on our attitudes towards women's health, and female patients are reaping the benefits in terms of better outcomes. There is still much work to be done, but we are at last seeing a positive recognition of specific female health issues that for so many years remained a neglected field of medicine. Women now have gynaecologists, breast surgeons and menopause experts; there is national screening for breast and cervical cancer, and better access to ante- and post-natal care (both physical and mental). Of course, all these developments should be welcomed, but where are the equivalent advances in the treatment of men's health issues?

There is no such thing as a 'men's health consultant' in the NHS. It could be argued that this is because you can't have a gynaecologist who is interested in male illnesses, and that practically every medical specialist looks at his or her own patients individually, takes into account male risk factors and acts accordingly. But, in practice, improving health outcomes for men requires more than just taking their gender into account when formulating a treatment plan. There are no national prostate or testicular cancer screening programmes, and conditions such as testosterone deficiency and erectile dysfunction are under-recognised by the public and poorly understood by many health professionals. Finally, mental health remains a taboo subject for the majority of men, as we are still expected to fit into a cultural narrative that insists we need to be tough and 'man up'.

To make matters worse, most men visit the doctor only when they have a problem; the concept of preventative medicine, or going for a check-up or a health 'MOT', remains a sign of weakness or failure. I still have patients who boast about not seeing a doctor for 20 years, as if this is a good thing. But with so many aspects of male health being poorly understood, we must ask the question, 'Do most men know how overlooked their health is?'

My interest in men's health developed by chance rather than design. I have always led a healthy lifestyle, and I have trained at a gym since I was seventeen. This was something I picked up from my father, who, despite being in his seventies, is still able to play football with my son and remains more fit and healthy than the majority of his peers. When I worked in A&E and started my job as a GP, many men would come to see me rather than my colleagues, as they felt that, as a young and fit man myself, I would be receptive to their personal problems and probably more able to help. It did not take long for me to realise that I was seeing the majority of erectile dysfunction and post-traumatic stress disorder patients as well as men who were struggling with obesity, fitness or concerns over their general well-being.

Although flattering, I found that while I was able to treat simple problems, cases of a more complex nature proved difficult, as there was no one I could refer to for help; for example, testosterone deficiency could be referred to the local endocrinologist (hormone specialist), but it was only one aspect of many hormonal problems they would deal with and, as such, many patients felt that their treatment remained suboptimal. Growing increasingly frustrated with the lack of support and my inability to help patients in need, I decided to find the answers to their problems myself. Over the next few years, I attended urology lectures, signed up for sexual medicine conferences, and spoke to endo-crinologists and psychologists. I wrote articles for medical journals and taught junior doctors about specific aspects of men's health. As my knowledge and confidence in this area continued to grow, I started to see men from further afield, and I gradually realised that there is a general lack of understanding about men's bodies, as well as a reluctance among most men to look after their health proactively. It was for this reason that I decided to write *Man Alive*.

The aim of this book is to provide a comprehensive guide

to health for men. Chapters 1 to 3 address the broadest aspects of men's health, including testosterone deficiency and the concept of male menopause, cardiovascular problems and wellness, and mental health. Despite the obvious importance of these areas for all men, they remain poorly understood and largely under-recognised. The second half of the book, Chapters 4 to 8, covers specifically male anatomical and physiological issues, including erectile dysfunction, baldness, beards, testicular problems, and prostate disease – all areas that men find difficult to discuss. These chapters offer detailed advice on symptoms and signs to look out for, how to self-examine, and when to consider seeing a doctor. Finally, now that you have decided to take an active interest in improving your health, Chapter 9 provides a no-nonsense guide to starting your journey towards a better quality of life.

Interspersed with every factual chapter are a range of case studies, all based on real scenarios I have encountered at some point in my career, although I have changed identifying details to ensure confidentiality. Some of the stories are comedic, others tragic, but all of them highlight a specific aspect of men's health and why we need to approach it differently.

Bad health is not inevitable for men. The key to improving the situation is to empower men with the knowledge they need to understand their own bodies and minds. By doing so, we will improve health outcomes and finally start to close the health gender gap.

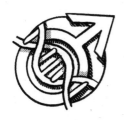

CASE STUDY

Are you John?

John was 42 years old and worked in a senior position at a bank. He was married with two children – a five-year-old daughter and a ten-year-old son. His daughter was energetic and devoted to her dad, constantly wanting to spend time with him whenever he was home. His son was similarly active and wanted John to be involved in all his daily sporting activities. John had been happily married for 15 years and loved his wife deeply. He knew that his life was comfortable, and he was grateful for all he had achieved.

John considered himself to be fit and healthy. He had played football and rugby in his twenties, and still prided himself on his fitness and sporting prowess; however, as time went by, work became busier, his children placed greater demands on his free time and he started to feel that he had no time to himself in the way he used to. He accepted that he was more sedentary and less physically active than he had been in his youth, and that he spent much longer at work and often ate badly during the day. As a consequence, by the time he got home, he was tired and hungry, and the last thing he wanted to do – especially with both of the children wanting his attention – was spend more time out of the house exercising. He would collapse on the sofa, play briefly with the kids, and only much later, when they had gone to bed, finally sit down to eat his one proper meal of the day.

Recently, John had noticed that he was developing a paunch

around his waist. His wife had noticed, too, especially when John had to buy trousers with a larger waist for the first time since they met. John shrugged this off and pointed out that he was now in his forties so he could hardly be expected to look the same as when they first met. In addition to his expanding waistband, he was finding it increasingly difficult to keep up with the pace and energy of his children. Again, though, he was relaxed about this, saying to himself: *No man in his forties should attempt to compare himself with a ten-year-old.*

John justified his larger trousers and insidious tiredness as just natural consequences of getting older – the inevitable lot of every 40-something. John had also recently started enjoying the taste of red wine. He had been a beer drinker in his twenties and thirties, but he now enjoyed a few glasses of red wine with his evening meal. It was something he and his wife did together, and it allowed John to unwind and talk about his day. He comically boasted to his friends that at the end of every two weeks his recycling bin was the heaviest in the street because of all the bottles it contained. He knew he was probably drinking too much but told himself it wasn't excessive, and it afforded him that quality time with this wife that he needed. Sadly, though, in marked contrast to when they were younger, a few drinks did not lead to anything more exciting. After dinner, John's wife would usually 'slip into something more comfort-able', a literal description of her pyjamas. Thereafter, they would spend an hour independently checking their phones in bed before John would fall asleep, hoping to wake refreshed the next day.

Unfortunately, John never woke refreshed. He always felt tired, but told himself this was normal because he was working hard and, after all, he was in his forties. He had tried to go to the gym, and even bought a fitness book that promised to 'change your life in eight weeks'; however, had given up after only two, and defensively explained to his wife that work didn't allow him to exercise as much as the book required. It was around this time that he caught himself being snappy with his wife and kids, and even his work colleagues said in jest – or so John thought – that he needed a holiday. Unfortunately, two weeks in the sun didn't really change anything. John was just as tired as he had been before, and he was unable to achieve an orgasm on the few occasions when he and his wife tried to have sex. This actually made things worse between them, so John felt the best thing to do was not to try having sex again for a while. He eventually went to his doctor to discuss his irritability and tiredness.

'What do you expect?' his doctor asked. 'You're working way too hard, you don't do any exercise, and you drink too much.'

It was precisely the response John had expected, and he told his GP that he was only really there because his wife had insisted. He just felt he had to tick the box.

'Okay,' said his GP, 'I tell you what. I'll arrange some blood tests to make sure you're not anaemic and your liver's okay, but I expect everything will be normal. Tiredness is such as common problem – nearly one in ten patients come in with it and most of the time it's all just down to lifestyle and getting older.'

Unsurprisingly, the blood tests came back normal, and following another appointment, John was given some antidepressants, told to address his lifestyle and come back in a few months' time. He took the medication for only three weeks as it made him feel worse than ever. He also decided that there was no point in booking another appointment as the problem was obvious: he was simply getting old.

A few weeks later, John was forced to endure yet another

torturous dinner with his wife's sister and her husband. He had been tormented by his sister-in-law's graphic descriptions of her menopausal symptoms for months now and while trying to feign interest, John sat thinking to himself *If I have to hear about your lack of sex drive and dry vagina one more time . . .*

Then it hit him. A couple of days earlier, on a particularly irritating train journey, he had started to read a newspaper article about low testosterone, but the stupid title, 'Manopause', had put him off. Now, though, the more he heard his sister-in-law prattle on about her night sweats and lack of desire, he felt a light bulb of recognition switching on in his head. He too had become more irritable, forgetful and generally grumpy. His body had definitely changed to such an extent that he hated the way he looked compared with just five years ago. He couldn't remember the last time he had wanted to have sex. He had even suffered a few night sweats, but he had put them down to the booze.

Eventually, after googling all his symptoms, John booked an appointment to have his testosterone checked, and found that his level was far lower than would be expected for a man of his age. He was diagnosed with testosterone deficiency, and through a process of medication, coupled with some major lifestyle changes, he gradually started to feel more like himself again. Over the next six months, he stopped drinking during the week, played sports with his son, read to his daughter and stopped napping after dinner. He was able to throw away his large trousers and even managed a romantic weekend away with his wife. For the first time in years, John actually had a morning erection and felt refreshed when he woke up each day.

For years, John had thought he was just getting old, not least because everyone he spoke to, and everything he did, served to confirm his suspicions that his symptoms were normal for a man of his age. After all, why would any 40-year-old expect to be able to do what they could do when they were 20? He had simply accepted his fate. But his problems were not just due to age and lifestyle. He was a victim of the silent, forgotten epidemic of male testosterone deficiency. And there are thousands of 'Johns', across the world who are struggling to understand why their lives have become so difficult.

CHAPTER 1

Testosterone Deficiency – The Forgotten Epidemic

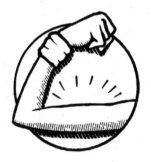

Almost as soon as I reached 40, people started saying, 'It's because you're getting old', 'You can't do that at your age' and 'Well, it's not like you're 20 any more' – with reference to a range of physical activities I undertake. Although often said in jest, there is some truth behind these comments. There is widespread acceptance that it is normal for men to lose their sex drive, get fat and take naps after dinner once they reach their late thirties, due to a combination of age itself, hectic jobs, the demands of young families and a general decline in the 'me time' we had when we were younger.

Getting old is more than just chronological

Although there is no doubt that ageing, coupled with daily pressures and commitments, will have an impact on our ability to achieve what we could physically 20 years ago, for a significant number of men, the decline in health and wellness they feel is not just a result of a busy work–life balance, but an under-recognised, poorly understood and potentially devastating medical condition: low testosterone. Often fobbed off as simply a consequence of age, it results in men being left to suffer unnecessarily with a variety of symptoms that affect their physical and mental health, harm their relationships and often contribute to serious illness. This is the impact that low testosterone is having on thousands of men, many of whom do not even realise that anything is wrong.

What does testosterone do?

Everyone has heard of testosterone, and most of us have a reasonable idea of what it does. In fact, it is probably the most widely discussed hormone: it dominates male-health forums; it is a crucial selling tactic for supplement companies; and no matter what health magazines we read, we are bombarded with ways to 'boost' it. It is almost always mentioned in relation to fitness or virility, but, but in reality, testosterone does much more than simply make our muscles bigger.

Testosterone is the main sex hormone in males. As boys enter puberty, it is the release of testosterone that is responsible for the characteristics that make us men, such as a deeper voice, the growth of pubic and facial hair, increased muscle mass and sexual function. But under the surface, it also affects our bodies in many other ways from altering our metabolism, blood pressure, cholesterol, cardiovascular function and bone density. Meanwhile, in the brain, it stimulates our sex drive, enhances both aggression and concentration, affects our emotions, and even our ability to think and form memories.

In men, testosterone is produced and regulated through an intricate process that starts with the hypothalamus gland in the brain, and ends in the testes. As we enter puberty, our testicles do not simply start pumping out unregulated amounts of testosterone, as this would have catastrophic effects on our bodies and put our overall health at risk. Instead, our bodies have evolved a sophisticated feedback loop that carefully regulates the amount of testosterone we produce daily: our hypothalamus stimulates another gland – the pituitary – to release luteinising hormone, which in turn stimulates the testicles to release testosterone. The circulating testosterone is then detected by the hypothalamus gland and the feedback loop is complete. Unfortunately, while this is a very effective way to determine the level of testosterone our bodies need, it is also highly sensitive and is affected by a range of diseases, medications, the food we eat and also by age itself. Even a brief interference in this pathway, such as a stress response brought on by a common cold, will produce a temporary dip in testosterone production. It should come as no surprise, then, that chronic medical conditions, such as obesity, type-2 diabetes or even heavy alcohol intake, can have a persistent negative impact on this feedback loop, and will result in a persistent drop in testosterone production. Eventually this results in the onset of symptoms, and the development of the medical condition testosterone deficiency.

What is testosterone deficiency?

The medical term for testosterone deficiency (TD) is male hypogonadism, but it has also been dubbed the 'male menopause', 'andropause' or 'manopause'. The effects of severely low testosterone have been known for centuries on account of the altered behaviour and absent secondary sexual characteristics of castrated boys. A eunuch could continue to sing soprano, would be physically less dominant, and would not pose a sexual threat to their lord's mistresses. Nowadays, although there are some genetic disorders and diseases that can result in a total absence of testosterone, the condition is exceedingly rare. Virtually all of these men are diagnosed early on in life and they are put on appropriate treatment before their symptoms become severe. By contrast, moderate testosterone deficiency is not only much more common – with studies suggesting a prevalence of between 2.1 and 11.8 per cent among middle-aged men[1] – but often undiagnosed. This could equate to nearly 2 million men in the United Kingdom alone.

Testosterone levels naturally climb during our twenties and peak at around the age of 30. Thereafter, the level of production decreases by about 1 per cent a year.

Consequently, in theory, it should be possible to predict the age at which all men will become testosterone deficient. Unfortunately, though, like so many aspects of the human body, the development of TD is not that simple. Peak levels of testosterone differ from person to person, and lifestyle factors, such as diet, exercise and obesity, speed up or slow down the rate at which we lose our testosterone. But the most unusual feature seen in TD is that not all men with low levels of testosterone develop symptoms, and it is not obvious why.

As far as we know, race and ethnicity have no direct influence on testosterone levels, although the prevalence of TD does seem to vary according to the general health of a population; for example, it seems to be more common in countries with poor access to good nutrition. On the other hand, it is also prevalent in countries with high levels of obesity. As reflected by the variation in estimated population prevalence noted above, one of the biggest challenges in treating TD is obtaining a true measure of just how many people suffer with it. Not only are we faced with trying to diagnose a medical problem that commonly mimics the normal aspects of ageing, but many men are not even aware that the condition even exists.

Might I have testosterone deficiency?

One of the biggest challenges in diagnosing TD is that its symptoms vary from person to person, with milder cases resulting in little more than tiredness, decreased sex drive, grumpiness or irritability, and with struggles to keep weight off and to stay fit. It is easy to see how any or all of these symptoms might be misinterpreted as consequences of working too hard or just getting old; however, as levels of testosterone continue to drop, the effects on our health, both physically and mentally, become more obvious. The illustration below shows some of the main differences between a man with a healthy testosterone level and someone suffering with the effects of low testosterone.

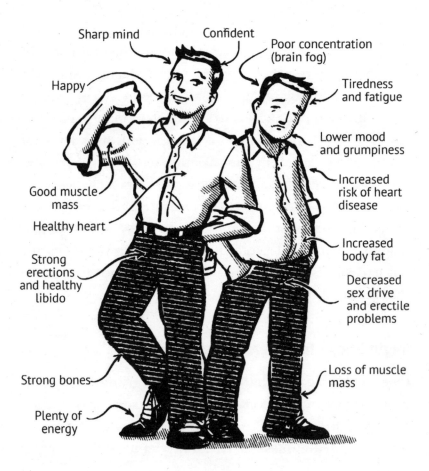

Sharp mind

Confident

Poor concentration (brain fog)

Happy

Tiredness and fatigue

Lower mood and grumpiness

Good muscle mass

Increased risk of heart disease

Healthy heart

Strong erections and healthy libido

Increased body fat

Decreased sex drive and erectile problems

Strong bones

Loss of muscle mass

Plenty of energy

As testosterone levels continue to drop, sufferers develop more advanced symptoms including those shown below.

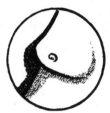

Development
of male breasts
(gynaecomastia)

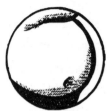

Significant
central obesity
and a paunch

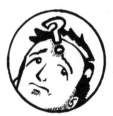

Memory
problems and
depression

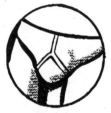

Reduction
in penis and
testicular size

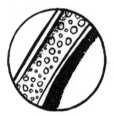

Decreased bone
density and
osteoporosis

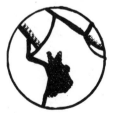

Night
sweats

Because the signs of TD are often vague and sometimes non-specific, it can be hard for patients and doctors alike to determine whether someone is suffering from low testosterone or a different medical condition with similar symptoms. With that in mind, the Androgen Deficiency in Ageing Males (ADAM) questionnaire was devised in 2000 to aid in the diagnosis of TD. The ten questions are quite broad, and although a high score does not prove that the patient is suffering from TD, a low score is quite effective at ruling it out.

The Androgen Deficiency in Ageing Males (ADAM) Questionnaire

1. Do you have a decrease in libido (sex drive)?   ☐ Yes ☐ No

2. Do you lack energy?   ☐ Yes ☐ No

3. Do you have a decrease in strength or endurance?   ☐ Yes ☐ No

4. Have you lost height?   ☐ Yes ☐ No

5. Have you noticed a decreased enjoyment of life?   ☐ Yes ☐ No

6. Are you sad and/or grumpy?   ☐ Yes ☐ No

7. Are your erections less strong?   ☐ Yes ☐ No

8. Have you noticed a recent deterioration in your ability to play sports?   ☐ Yes ☐ No

9. Do you fall asleep after dinner?   ☐ Yes ☐ No

10. Have you noticed a deterioration in your work performance?   ☐ Yes ☐ No

If you answer yes to question 1 or 7, or any three other questions, you might be suffering from low testosterone.

If the symptoms of TD were not enough to make us alarmed, the effects of low testosterone inside our bodies are potentially more serious. TD sufferers are at an increased risk of developing obesity, heart disease, high blood pressure and cholesterol, osteoporosis (reduced bone density) and memory impairment.[2] Furthermore, Diabetes UK estimates that approximately 25 per cent of all male patients with type-2 diabetes have lower than normal levels of testosterone.

What causes low testosterone?

In the UK, most cases of TD are due to age, obesity, type-2 diabetes or a combination of the three. But the additional potential causes of TD are so wide-ranging that we often fail to realise just how many other aspects of our health, lifestyle, or general wellness can also impact on our testosterone pathway.

Common conditions that can result in low testosterone		
Problems affecting the body	Medicines	Lifestyle factors
Ageing	Opiate painkillers (codeine, morphine)	Cannabis
Obesity	Antifungals	Obesity
Type-2 diabetes	Some diabetic medicines	Type-2 diabetes

Common conditions that can result in low testosterone		
Problems affecting the body	Medicines	Lifestyle factors
High blood pressure	Diuretics (water tablets)	Smoking
Liver disease	Chemotherapy and other cancer treatments	Alcohol
Chronic kidney disease	Anti-inflammatory steroids (prednisolone)	Lack of sleep
Lung disease, including asthma, chronic bronchitis and emphysema	Certain mental health drugs	Lack of exercise
Underactive thyroid	Possibly statins	Stress
Genetic conditions		
Testicular torsion (twisting of the testicle)		
Cancer		

Although this list may appear long, this is intentional to illustrate just how many external factors can have an impact on our ability to produce optimal levels of testosterone. And many other chronic inflammatory conditions and medications might also affect testosterone production. Even environmental factors and certain occupations have been linked to a reduction in levels, possibly as a result of exposure to chemicals that have oestrogenic properties, such as certain pesticides and a variety of household cleaning products. But while this link has been proposed, the true connection between environmental oestrogens and our own testosterone production has yet to be confirmed. With such a wide range of other factors potentially impacting on our testosterone levels, it is unsurprising that more and more men are coming forward to be tested.

I would strongly advise any man who thinks he might have low testosterone to have his levels checked by an appropriately trained doctor.

If you are going to check your testosterone level, do it properly

Testosterone production follows a circadian rhythm, which means that our levels peak in the early hours of the morning and tend to decline later in the day. This is the reason why men with healthy levels of testosterone experience those occasionally inconvenient morning erections, although this event doesn't necessarily occur daily even if normal levels of testosterone are released. Consequently, if you are going to have a blood test to check your testosterone level, it is crucial to make sure it is performed in the early morning, as blood tests taken in the afternoon will almost certainly yield an inaccurate result. There is one exception to this rule: anyone who does regular shift work should have the test done about three hours after waking, whenever that might be.

Approximately 60 per cent of testosterone is bound to a protein in our blood known as sex hormone binding globulin (SHBG), while a further 38 per cent is bound to a variety of other proteins. This means that in reality, only about 2 per cent of the testosterone that circulates in our blood is active at any one time. It is this 'free' testosterone that should always be measured during blood tests because the other 98 per cent, while potentially available for the body to use, is not biologically active. Many factors can increase or decrease the levels of SHBG and the other proteins that bind to testosterone, so if you strongly suspect that you have TD but your test results suggest everything is fine, make sure that the lab measured your 'free' rather than your 'total' testosterone level.

For many years, another big problem in diagnosing testosterone deficiency was that individual countries, clinics and scientists disagreed over what constitutes the normal range of testosterone for a fit and healthy man. This seemingly straightforward task is actually extremely complicated because in addition to varying considerably both during the day and from one day to the next, testosterone levels are affected by countless external factors, such as diet, exercise and sexual activity. Furthermore, a level of testosterone that causes one person to feel low might be completely normal for someone else. Hence, two equally reputable clinics could reach very different conclusions when analysing a single blood test, depending on their particular definition of 'low testosterone'. Perhaps the only way to achieve a truly accurate, objective diagnosis of TD would be to measure every man's testosterone level on his thirtieth birthday and use that as his personal baseline value for the rest of his life. Unfortunately, such a scheme is neither practical nor realistic.

In 2017, however, the British Society of Sexual Medicine finally provided some clarity on the subject of TD when it adopted the International Society for Sexual Medicine's guidelines on 'normal' levels of testosterone,[3] which suggest that 'total' testosterone should be in the region of 12–30nmol/l (or 346ng/dl) whereas 'free' testosterone should exceed 225pmol/l.[4] These benchmarks are undoubtedly useful as they eliminate the problem of individual clinics setting their own baseline levels, and it is now generally accepted that any patient who meets them does not require testosterone replacement therapy (with only rare exceptions).

What, though, of patients who fall below the 12nmol/l threshold? What sort of level should they hope to achieve through treatment? For example, does a man of 35 need more testosterone than a man in his sixties? Actually, the most recent research suggests that a minimum of 15nmol/l is sufficient for all men, regardless of age. And the really good news is that this level, and the associated health benefits, can be achieved and maintained through testosterone replacement therapy.

The evolutionary advantage of low testosterone

As mentioned earlier, testosterone production naturally declines by about 1 per cent a year after the age of 30. Therefore, although some of the consequences can be mitigated by frequent exercise, a good diet and a healthy lifestyle, every middle-aged man is still fighting nature's attempt to make him impotent. We tend to think of this process as a bad thing – either disease related or just a by-product of our bodies starting to fail as we age. But what if the gradual decline in testosterone production is actually a positive evolutionary adaptation that has helped the human species by creating generations of wise, placid grandfathers?[5]

High levels of testosterone are associated with increased aggression, greater sex drive and riskier behaviour. Therefore, some scientists theorise that nature reduces our testosterone later in life specifically to blunt some of our more perilous impulses, and by doing so improves our chances of living longer and helping to raise the next generation. After all, no one wants a grandfather who is constantly trying to have sex and starting fights. In many ways, this is a counterpart to the so-called grandmother hypothesis, which suggests that menopause is a valuable evolutionary process that allows older women to focus on caring for their grandchildren.

As it is inevitable that our testosterone declines as we age, we have to ask ourselves if we are happy to accept what nature has decided is our destiny. Or should we fight against our DNA? The comparison with female hormone replacement therapy (HRT) becomes increasingly pertinent once we start thinking along these lines. Until very recently, menopause was considered a natural aspect of ageing, and the life-altering symptoms and discomfort that many women experience were dismissed as normal or were trivialised. Menopause was certainly not viewed as a serious medical problem; indeed, some doctors still have that attitude towards it even today. Clearly, HRT is not for everyone, but to my mind every woman should at least be given the choice. And the same consideration should be given to men with low levels of testosterone.

We can only hypothesise as to whether evolution wants us to grow old gracefully, increasingly fat and impotent but non-threatening and calm. But whatever our genes have in store for us, we are lucky enough to live in an age when we do not have to accept age for what it is. We might not need or want to take testosterone supplements or HRT, but we should have the option to maximise both the quality and the quantity of our lives.

How do you treat low testosterone?

Many of the men who are diagnosed with TD assume that this automatically means starting testosterone replacement therapy. But this should be the last, not the first, course of action. The testosterone supplementation industry is huge, and many suppliers appeal directly to a public that is desperate to feel better. Global sales of medical testosterone replacement products already exceed £1.35 billion per year, and their powerful marketing campaigns are designed to convince sufferers that a low testosterone level can be fixed only through testosterone replacement.

In reality, testosterone replacement therapy (TRT) should be prescribed only once all other possible treatments have been explored; for example, one should always consider if any underlying medical issues or medications have triggered a decline in testosterone production. In addition, it is important to look at any lifestyle factors that could be contributing to a reduction in levels. Health measures should always be optimised to see if testosterone production can be improved naturally.

The importance of lifestyle factors in TD is often downplayed because changing your habits does not sell any drugs or make any companies rich. Moreover, addressing them is far from easy. I have had many patients who have specifically requested TRT on the grounds that they do not have the time to exercise or the wherewithal to eat better. But a drug is never an adequate substitute for living a healthier lifestyle. There are many ways you can boost your testosterone production naturally – here are some of the best.

Diet and supplements

Obesity and TD are intrinsically linked: obese men are more likely to have low testosterone, and men with low testosterone are more likely to become obese. The mechanism through which the two are connected is multifactorial, and this can make reducing body fat in the presence of reduced testosterone even more challenging, as it is a negative cycle that becomes increasingly hard to break. But the benefits of losing weight cannot be overstated: in obese patients, a 10 per cent reduction in body weight can increase the total testosterone level by up to 4nmol/l.

That said, the opposite is also true: being significantly underweight or rapidly reducing our daily food intake puts our bodies into a starvation state that suppresses testosterone production. If our energy expenditure considerably exceeds the number of calories we ingest, testosterone production can be put on hold to conserve energy for more vital functions.

From an evolutionary perspective this is a clever but selfish adaptation: our body prioritises its own survival over producing a hormone that will increase our chances of fathering the next generation. Practically, we should not even be thinking about having sex if we do not have enough food to survive.

The obvious take-home message is that we should aim for a normal weight that does not put unhealthy stress on our bodies by being either too heavy or too light. But there is more to the link between diet and testosterone production than simple body weight. A quick Google search results in dozens of websites featuring 'The best foods or supplements to boost testosterone levels'. It would be impossible to address all these here, but below I explain the impact (if any) of the most common recommendations. (Food's influence on our overall health and wellness is discussed in more detail in Chapter 2.)

Avoid high-calorie foods, such as sugar and fat. Generally this is true, as high-calorie foods tend to trigger a sudden decrease in testosterone level. Interestingly, though, this almost-immediate effect does not seem to be related to the level of insulin in the bloodstream, so further research is required to understand the link. In addition, excessive consumption of high-calorie foods usually leads to an increase in body fat, which suppresses testosterone production through a complex mechanism of increased insulin resistance and its impact on SHBG, higher levels of oestrogen, and an interruption of the testosterone feedback pathway. On the other hand, it should be remembered that very low-carb diets can push us into the starvation state mentioned above, so we should always aim for a balanced diet that includes some fat, some carbohydrate and some protein. (This is discussed in more detail in Chapter 2.)

Consume sufficient levels of healthy fats Just as we cannot function without any carbohydrates, the same is true for fat; however, most of us consume far too much of the wrong types of fat, which results in weight gain and a consequent suppression of testosterone production. Instead, we should eat more of the healthy fats that are found in nuts, oily fish (such as salmon and mackerel), avocados and whole eggs. We can even treat ourselves to the occasional piece of dark chocolate.

Tribulus terrestris, a weedy plant with small yellow flowers, has been advertised for decades as a natural testosterone-boosting supplement, and it is included in the majority of over-the-counter testosterone boosters. Sadly, though, there is little to no evidence that it increases testosterone production in humans. Furthermore, high levels are associated with liver toxicity.

Fenugreek is also touted as a testosterone booster due to its active component *furostanolic saponins*. Again, although it has been incorporated into over-the-counter products for many years, there is no good evidence that it has any positive effect in humans.

Vitamin D Over recent years, there has been increased interest in the role of vitamin D in treating everything from hormone imbalances to bowel cancer, and even coronavirus. In terms of TD, the evidence for the efficacy of vitamin D supplementation is mixed. Certainly, men with low vitamin D levels might suffer disruption to their hormonal pathways, but at present it is best to assume that exceeding the normal daily allowance will have no impact on testosterone production.

Zinc and selenium are both used in the optimisation of fertility and to enhance sperm production; however, when it comes to boosting testosterone, neither should be taken above the recommended daily allowance, as they are unlikely to increase production and may result in toxicity. Indeed, my advice is to avoid supplementation, as this is unlikely to do anything for your testosterone level. Instead, try to eat foods that contain naturally high levels of zinc and selenium, such as meat, shellfish, nuts, dairy and eggs.

Magnesium Interestingly, unlike many other minerals, magnesium supplementation does appear to have the potential to increase – or at least maximise – testosterone levels. This is because it is known to produce better-quality, deep sleep, which is not only essential for efficient testosterone production but it is also a safe, natural way to improve our overall wellness.

Physiologically, we cannot boost our testosterone above a maximum level that the human body is able to produce naturally. We can *maximise* our body's potential to produce testosterone by eating a healthy, balanced diet and maintaining an optimal body weight, but any product

that truly *boosted* testosterone would have to bypass our
normal physiology and act like an anabolic steroid. Put
simply, if *Tribulus terrestris* and fenugreek really increased
our testosterone levels, they would not be available in
health-food stores because they would be classified as
medical-grade drugs and would therefore require a prescription. Supplement manufacturers have not found a loophole
in the law that enables them to sell powerful testosterone-
boosting supplements directly to the public. Rather, they
have found a way to market products that just don't work.

Exercise

We all know that exercise is good for us. As well as increasing testosterone levels, it helps us to lose weight and releases
endorphins: natural chemicals produced by the pituitary
gland that make us feel good, combat stress and reduce
pain. For a long time, it has been assumed that weight-
lifting is the paramount testosterone-boosting exercise, but
is pumping iron really preferable to going for a run?

Research shows that lifting weights for 30 to 45 minutes
several times per week does indeed increase testosterone
production, but other forms of cardiovascular exercise,
especially those that involve short bursts of high activity
coupled with brief periods of recovery – the so-called high-
intensity interval training (HIIT) – can be equally effective.
It seems to be the intensity, rather than the particular type
of exercise, that is the crucial factor.

By contrast, both elite and recreational athletes who
compete in low-intensity, high-duration sports, such as

marathon running or long-distance cycling, can actually reduce their testosterone levels by pushing their bodies into a pseudo-starvation state. These athletes tend to function with very low body fat levels, and exercise at an intensity most of us will never achieve. However, a mild version of this effect can be seen in men who overtrain.

'Overtraining syndrome' is a process by which our efforts to exercise outweigh our ability to recover. We simply train too much. Symptoms of overtraining include loss of motivation to exercise further, combined with flu-like symptoms and perpetual fatigue, as well as poorer recovery. More importantly, overtraining results in a negative effect on our sex-hormone pathway, and produces a measurable decline in testosterone production. This phenomenon is not unusual and is commonly seen in many professional and amateur athletes. Fortunately, there is a simple remedy: take a training holiday. The optimum length of this holiday depends on a variety of factors, including age, level of fitness and type of exercise. A week is usually sufficient, but it's advisable to continue to refrain from all exercise until you feel fully rested and symptom-free.

Sleep

We are told time and time again, that sleep is essential for our health, but it is also vital for testosterone production. Although this varies with age, ideally we need between seven and eight hours of sleep per night, and, most importantly, this should be uninterrupted sleep to make sure that we get the deep sleep required to produce a testosterone surge each morning. It is this early testosterone surge that is responsible for our morning erections. One study found that even over just a single week, reducing sleep to fewer than five hours a night reduced testosterone levels by 15 per cent.[6] Therefore, we should never underestimate just how important a good night's sleep is for our overall well-being.

Below are several ways to promote good sleep:

Set a routine If you take only one thing from this list, establishing a decent sleep routine is my most useful tip. Good sleep hygiene involves going to bed at the same time each day, avoiding caffeine for up to seven hours before bed, and getting into a bedtime routine so that your brain knows when it's time for sleep. This might mean having a bath, drinking a glass of milk or protein shake, or reading a book.

Get comfortable This sounds obvious, but sleeping on the couch is not conducive to good sleep; equally, a cheap bed disturbs sleep quality and can result in postural problems. It is worth buying the best bed that you can afford and trying it out in the showroom before purchasing it to be sure that you have the comfort and support that you need.

Keep your bedroom quiet When we sleep, our bodies continue to respond to external stimuli, so keeping the bedroom dark, cool and comfortable is essential for a good night's sleep.

Only use your bed for sex or sleeping. Although reading or doing a sudoku (for example), is fine, it is important not confuse what we do as our daytime activities with the process of trying to sleep. Therefore, brain-stimulating behaviours, such as eating or working just before we lie down, are likely to have detrimental effects on our association between our beds and sleep.

Avoid eating a large meal just before bed. Big meals require significant amounts of digestive effort, and in addition to being harder to metabolise (potentially resulting in greater fat storage), they also increase the chances of indigestion and acid reflux because we are lying flat with a large food bolus resting in our stomach.

Keep distractions out of the bedroom Don't put a television in the bedroom and keep tablets and other screens outside (but see box below). It is not so much the screens themselves that can be a problem, it's more that the stimulating effect of watching TV or checking social media makes it hard for our brains to relax.

You cannot build up sleep credits Sleeping longer one night will not reduce our need for sleep the next, and, sadly, a lie-in at the weekend won't repair bad sleeps during the week. Our bodies are not able to store extra sleep for later on, and our overall sleep requirement tends not to vary significantly on a day-to-day basis.

Are mobile phones really so bad?

It has been suggested that using mobile phones at bedtime could adversely affect sleep, and that idea has been quickly picked up and presented by the media because it is a simple concept and a highly sellable story; however, like a great deal of popular science, things are never that straightforward. The assumption here is that mobile phones not only act as a stimulus for our brain but that the blue light from the screen suppresses melatonin, the hormone responsible for our sleep pattern. Recently, however, this theory is being challenged, as more and more people find that they are able to sleep without difficulty, despite looking at their phones in bed. The most likely reason for this is that the blue light is not quite so detrimental to our sleep patterns as was first thought, and perhaps it is the content of what we see on our phones that affects our sleep rather than the screen itself. Therefore, if you do decide to use your phone in bed, perhaps the best approach is to make sure you read something relaxing, and not get tempted to answer work emails, get involved in political discussions on Facebook or Twitter, or watch scary movies. You could also set the night timer on your phone if you find it more comfortable to read in the evening, which automatically changes to a yellow light during the hours of darkness.

Stress management

Stressful events lead to the release of the hormone cortisol. Cortisol is essential for our bodies to function: we need it to keep our blood pressure up to a healthy level so that we can function, stay alert and awake, and maintain our blood-glucose levels. It also helps the body to fight infections. But cortisol is also an antagonist to testosterone.

During the course of human evolution, the fight-or-flight response that cortisol triggers has been crucial in helping us survive, because when danger threatens it primes the body to fight or run in the opposite direction. In the 21st century, however, most of us will never be chased by lions or need to fight a rhino. Our bodies, therefore, have become far more sensitive to other forms of stress. This can have a chronic detrimental effect on testosterone production. Although I will address anxiety in more detail in Chapter 3 on mental health, there are several simple ways in which we can reduce our daily stress levels to help to maintain a normal testosterone profile:

- Get more exercise. Of course, the amount of exercise required to reduce stress will vary from person to person and will also need to be amended based on whether the exercise is for fitness or intended only to improve mental health. But in terms of pure stress relief, even 20 minutes of exercise a day, away from computer screens, moving our bodies and spending time in nature, can be enough to reduce stress levels.
- Create a stress-free environment, especially before bed.
- Reduce caffeine intake from coffee and tea.
- Spend time with friends, family and your pets.
- Learn to say no! Having too much to do creates more stress.
- Find a mindfulness method that works for you: almost any form of meditation can help to reduce anxiety and negative thinking. One easy way to practise a simple form of meditation is to step away

from the stressful trigger, relax and take 10–30 slow,
deep breaths. Even this basic action can cause a near
immediate calming effect.
- Ignore your phone for the first hour of every day.

Sex

There is a lot of myth and superstition around the impact of
sexual activity (with or without a partner) on testosterone
production, and there is no doubt that the two are linked.
We know that higher levels of testosterone increase libido
and can affect orgasm, but does the opposite also apply?

The first thing to note is that our bodies do not differentiate between masturbating or having sexual intercourse
with someone, therefore the outcomes on testosterone production and other hormones are irrelevant to how orgasm
is achieved. The second thing to note is that when it comes
to testosterone secretion, evidence is conflicting. Although
some studies have shown that during sex, testosterone levels
transiently rise, they are often lowered again post-orgasm,
due to an increase in the hormone prolactin. (This is the
hormone responsible for breast-milk production in women,
but it also affects emotions and anxiety in both males and
females.) Overall, the studies have found that there is a zero
net gain in testosterone production; however, these studies
are almost always carried out in an unnatural environment
(a lab), and this might not represent the true hormonal patterns that we would experience when having sex.

Other studies have also found that short-term abstinence
does increase testosterone levels, with significant rises

measured at one week[7] and three weeks after sex.[8] There is also some evidence to suggest that prolonged abstinence of greater than 12 weeks has the opposite effect, because it is associated with reduced testosterone production. Both these observations make sense from an evolutionary perspective. In the first instance, the body has recently had sex, so it produces more testosterone in preparation to have more sex again and therefore to reproduce. If no sex is forthcoming, the body reduces its testosterone production, because it is not required for reproduction.

Medical treatment of TD: testosterone replacement therapy

For those men who have already tried everything they can naturally do to improve their testosterone levels, or for those who might have underlying medical problems that they cannot alter, testosterone replacement therapy (TRT) can be a highly effective treatment. The principle of TRT is simple: it literally replaces the testosterone that is lacking with the aim of therapy to raise levels back to normal. It is worth emphasising this point, however: the only purpose of TRT is to correct a deficiency. We are not trying to make super-humans, and irrespective of the wishes of individuals who might want to abuse the drug, doctors have a moral and ethical responsibility to treat only those men who have a confirmed testosterone deficiency. I have written this specifically because I have had requests from numerous patients who are already abusing anabolic steroids who have asked if I would 'monitor them' to make sure that they are safe. This is an oxymoron; you cannot abuse a drug to take the body to unnatural levels and expect to stay healthy. Unsurprisingly, when my answer is that I am happy to help, but the first thing we need to do is reduce the current medication dose by 100 per cent, these men go elsewhere.

In general, TRT is well tolerated by almost all men, and, if used correctly, it is a safe and easy to drug to administer. Furthermore, by using it for the correct patient, TRT can be a life-changing medicine that betters not only the quality of life for an individual but actually improves the risk profile for other diseases such as heart disease, high blood pressure, high cholesterol, osteoporosis and many others.

TRT forms of medication

If you do decide to take testosterone replacement, there are several ways it can be administered. Methods include oral tablets, topical gels and creams, and short- or long-acting injections. Outside the UK, there are also patches, pellets, or even a form of treatment that involves rubbing a gel onto the gums. Depending on which clinic you visit, you might find that individual doctors advocate a specific form of treatment or therapy as being better than all the others (such as micro-injection techniques), but in truth there is no right answer or best treatment. All men are different – the best form of therapy is the one that suits you.

What to expect from TRT

TRT is a long-term treatment that exerts different effects on the body over time. Even within the first few weeks of starting treatment patients commonly report feeling more energised and less fatigued, and they display better focus and mental clarity. At about three weeks men often start to report improved sexual function, including better erections and sexual desire, but the true benefits to erectile function continue for up to six months due to changes in metabolism and vascular blood supply. By that stage the beneficial effects of TRT on erectile function are likely to have been optimised. In addition, within the first few months of treatment, patients often report improvements in mood and mental health, and the brain fog they have experienced starts to lift and they feel that they have a better quality of life. Overall, the benefits of TRT tend to affect men at different rates, however, and it is therefore important to give each patient a trial of six months' therapy before deciding if the treatment is right for them.

Is TRT safe?

There are many misconceptions around TRT, the most common of which is that it can increase the chances of developing prostate cancer. This is completely false. Testosterone is needed for healthy prostate function and development, and although complete removal of testosterone would make it very hard to develop prostate cancer, there is no evidence that men treated with TRT have an increased risk of developing either a benign large prostate (known as benign prostatic hyperplasia – BPH),[9] or have an increased risk of prostate cancer.[10] The key is to rule out, wherever possible, any pre-existing prostate disease prior to starting therapy. If there is any suspicion of either prostate or breast cancer, TRT should not be initiated, as this could effectively cause the undiagnosed cancer to grow rapidly or spread, because it is usually highly testosterone sensitive.

Much like the worries over TRT and prostate cancer, there have also been incorrect links made between TRT and the development of heart disease. In fact, the opposite is true. Men with high blood pressure, high cholesterol, type-2 diabetes or other conditions that increase their risk of heart disease, are more likely to also suffer with low testosterone, and there is now good evidence that getting testosterone levels back to normal can actually reduce the risk of suffering a heart attack.

The use of TRT is not entirely risk-free however, and although when used correctly the risks are low, it is important that patients are monitored regularly by their doctor. Although some of the milder side effects include acne, a raised red blood cell count or even ankle swelling, probably the most important side effect to be aware of when considering TRT is that it results in a degree of infertility. This is a really important factor to consider before starting therapy in any patient who might want to have a family. For these men, I suggest either postponing therapy until after conceiving, freezing sperm to put it into storage, or coming off therapy for at least three to six months before trying for a child, as this usually allows sperm production to become active again.

What should I do if I think I might have low testosterone?

If you have read this chapter and think you might be suffering with low testosterone, the first thing to do is look at a testosterone scoring system, such as the ADAM questionnaire on page 20. If you score highly on this, or you think you might have low testosterone anyway, before you embark on blood tests or other investigations, you might wish to look at lifestyle factors and decide whether there is anything you can do to improve your testosterone levels naturally. If you have already addressed these factors, or you have other medical problems, or there are other barriers that mean you cannot improve your testosterone, the next step is to speak to a doctor.

I strongly advise against simply ordering testosterone blood tests online without speaking to a doctor first. It is important that a health professional with an understanding of male health takes your history, listens to your symptoms and then decides which blood tests are appropriate to suit your individual case. If you simply order a testosterone blood test, it might either falsely reassure you that your levels are normal or it could miss another disease that could have been diagnosed and treated had the correct tests been performed.

Even if your testosterone levels are shown as low, it is still relatively common to be denied treatment on the NHS due to the fact that different regions set their own reference range for what an acceptable testosterone level should be. This range is always far lower than what would be required for a formal diagnosis of testosterone deficiency, and sadly it is usually only men with severely low levels of testosterone that are treated through NHS clinics; however, this should not dissuade you from seeking treatment, but it might mean that you have to obtain therapy through a private medical clinic.

The future of TRT

I believe that the way we approach TRT and low testosterone in men is similar to the way HRT for female menopause was perceived by many women five or ten years ago. It has taken a tremendous amount of research and effort by clinicians and support groups for HRT to be taken seriously after initial scares and negative media hype, and I hope that TRT might be heading along a similar route.

As we live longer, and the numbers of men with obesity, type-2 diabetes and other testosterone-suppressing conditions increase, we need to stop thinking of testosterone deficiency as a normal consequence of ageing. It is only when we approach TRT as being more than a drug used by bodybuilders or trivialised as a quirky remedy for middle-aged tiredness that we will make significant gains in improving the quality of life and reducing mortality for men with low testosterone.

Summary

- Testosterone is essential for making us men.
- It gives us energy, concentration, sex drive and muscle mass, and it keeps body fat down.
- In addition, it also improves our mental health and keeps our bones healthy, and it improves blood pressure, cholesterol and other markers of cardiovascular disease.
- Testosterone deficiency might affect up to 2 million men in the UK.
- Symptoms are often confused with the natural process of ageing, and so they can be hard to detect.
- Multiple lifestyle factors and medical conditions can adversely affect testosterone levels.
- Testing is easy, via a simple blood test, once you have consulted with a doctor.

Awareness is empowering: not everyone with low testosterone needs treatment, and by following the lifestyle measures suggested in this chapter, most men will be able to increase or optimise their natural testosterone production.

For those men who have already improved their lifestyles with little or no effect, if used correctly, testosterone replacement therapy remains a safe and highly effective treatment.

Our bodies go through numerous changes as we grow older. For many men, these changes are perceived as a normal part of the ageing process, but it is not true for every man. It is only by being aware of how low testosterone can adversely affect our bodies and minds that we will be able to treat this problem effectively and improve health outcomes for those many men affected.

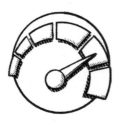

CASE STUDY

The man who could not lose weight

I first met Gareth and his wife about four years ago after he had been invited to attend the practice for a health check. He had declined previous invitations but had reached the age of 50, and decided that it would be useful for him to have a health assessment done to prove to his wife that he was still fit and healthy, and could continue for another 20 years without seeing a doctor. Unfortunately for Gareth, his review had uncovered not only raised cholesterol and high blood pressure, but also that he was classed as obese. As a result, the nurse had asked him to see me to address these issues, as he needed a radical lifestyle change and might also require medication.

When I met Gareth, he brought his wife in with him, but oddly failed to introduce her and ignored her for the entire consultation. After introducing myself, I did my usual spiel about what high blood pressure and high cholesterol meant and how this relates to heart disease and stroke. We also discussed how Gareth's weight was a contributing factor to his overall health. As this is a relatively common conversation I have with patients, I find it is really important not to appear too paternal in my approach, and I always try to stress the reversible nature of many of the problems the patient has presented with. With some positive encouragement and motivation, we might get away with not having to prescribe medication at all, but this usually requires significant lifestyle changes to be made. Oddly, his response was one of simple denial.

'No, I don't agree with you,' Gareth said in a matter-of-fact tone. 'I hardly eat anything and I'm still active. I walk the dog every day and I don't snack. This is just my genes.'

It is quite common for people who are overweight to be frustrated by those who appear to eat far more than them but remain thin. But even if genetics might have dealt someone an unfair hand, we can all improve our lifestyle and make better choices for our health. I attempted to highlight how much diet was contributing to Gareth's current medical situation, but once again he disagreed, blaming his wife for feeding him too much. This felt rather uncomfortable with her sitting next to him. After another few minutes of trying to impress the relevance of diet and weight on overall health, I needed to draw the consultation to a close, so we agreed that as a compromise, Gareth would keep a food diary of everything he ate for the next two weeks, and then come back and see me with the results. I also asked him to photograph his meals, as this often gives a better idea of portion size. Two weeks later Gareth re-entered my consultation room with his beleaguered wife a few paces behind him. As he marched in, he tossed something at me dismissively. 'There you go,' he said, before sitting and folding his arms in triumphant defiance.

It was his food diary, and as I looked through, it was obvious that he had written the bare minimum. Pages were populated with entries such as:

Tuesday

Breakfast	Lunch	Dinner
Piece of fruit and black coffee	Sandwich – brown bread Ham Apple	Stir-fry chicken, noodles and vegetables

Every page in the diary contained the same sparse and minimal content. After firstly clarifying that he hadn't suddenly changed his diet (which he said he hadn't), I explained that this diary was not really what I had asked for.

'I meant you write down *literally* everything you eat for the food diary, ideally with pictures. Otherwise it's really hard to get a true idea about what you're really eating,' I explained.

'It's what you asked for,' Gareth said dismissively.

'Okay,' I replied. 'So, assuming these are normal portion sizes, this is all you ate for a week?' (He had not bothered to complete two weeks' worth of the food diary.)

'Yeah, like I told you before, I don't each much,' he replied.

At this point I clarified that unless these portion sizes were actually three times the size of a normal portion, there was no way this was more than around 1,000 calories per day and could not account for Gareth's current body size.

'Well I don't know what to tell you, doc. That's just the way it is,' he protested. 'Maybe it's my thyroid?'

Almost all doctors have had patients query the effective functioning of their thyroid gland at some point in their lives when they have been either tired or overweight. But in men in particular, this is less commonly the case due to the genetic differences between the sexes. In an effort to try to keep Gareth on side, I asked if he would repeat the food diary, just for a week, but this time with pictures, and then come back and see me again in two weeks' time. He agreed, but made a rather juvenile eyebrow raise to his wife as if to highlight the futility of this proposal.

Gareth didn't come back as planned, but actually returned in six weeks as, apparently, he had been on holiday. This time he had photographed every dinner he had eaten for a week but no other foods. He had also put on 3 kilograms, but attributed this to his week away.

This time, I informed Gareth that whether he agreed with me or not, his body weight was unsafe and increasing. His blood pressure and cholesterol were reflections of this, and if he did not take action soon, he could end up having a heart attack or stroke. Refusing to try any specific diet plan, I suggested that whatever he eats, he should discard one quarter of the plate with each meal (as I had no real idea what his diet actually consisted of). I also explained that a 20-minute gentle walk with the dog was not the exercise his body needed, which had to be more intense and last longer. I asked Gareth to come back in three months for a blood test and review, at which point we would have to think about starting medication if things had not improved.

Six months passed before Gareth came back to see me. To be honest, I was surprised to see him at all based on our previous conversations, as I never thought he wanted to see me. I was not completely wrong though, as it turns out the only reason he had agreed to come in was that his repeat blood tests had shown worsening results. In addition to his existing medical problems, he had now developed type-2 diabetes.

As expected, he was full of excuses. He had injured his ankle so he couldn't walk the dog, he had tried to eat less but his conspiring wife had mercilessly kept serving him large portions, he had a sedentary job that took all day so there was no time to exercise and, most importantly, none of this was really Gareth's fault, as he didn't eat anything.

'What do you want me to do?' I asked. 'You clearly don't want to take my advice, and all your markers of health are getting worse. You need to be on medication now, but to be honest, like I've said before, this really comes down to you, and how much you want to help yourself.'

Gareth begrudgingly accepted medication for his blood pressure and cholesterol, he agreed to see the diabetic-nurse specialist, and once again we arranged to meet, this time in two weeks, to see how he was getting on. Unsurprisingly, he didn't show. I also noted that one month later he did not order his repeat medication, and I assumed he had chosen to stop taking it.

I had no further interaction with Gareth until one year later when I was informed via a hospital discharge letter that he had been recently admitted to the local cardiac unit having suffered a major heart attack. His cardiac disease had been so severe that he had spent two weeks in coronary intensive care and was lucky to be alive. Frustratingly, although not that unexpected, Gareth had repeatedly ignored the health advice given to him from our practice and had not once ordered the medication I had prescribed him. But what I found most puzzling, however, was that according to the letter, when Gareth arrived at hospital he denied having any other health problems and took no medication. This included high blood pressure and, astonishingly, his diagnosis of diabetes.

Gareth was discharged on six new medications and advised to attend his GP surgery for a review.

On receiving his letter, I phoned Gareth and left an answer-phone message asking him to make an appointment to see me. I also sent a formal letter to his house requesting him to come in so that we could review the medication started by the hospital but more to see how he was getting on. Gareth never attended and, once more, at the end of the month, his new repeat medications were never ordered.

Three months later, and nearly two years since I first met Gareth, out of the blue I received a letter from his wife, written on his behalf, asking if I would support his application for a Blue Badge for disabled parking. According to Gareth's wife, he could now only walk a few metres without getting out of breath and needed our support. In the letter, Gareth's wife stated that they both felt let down by the NHS, as no one had helped him with his health problems, in particular his heart and lungs.

Once again, I wrote to Gareth to ask him to come in and discuss his application or to at least make a phone appointment with me but, as always, he never replied. I never completed his Blue Badge application and I have not heard from him or his wife since. I will never know why he refused to take any responsibility for his health, but it was clear that even after he had been hospitalised and operated on, Gareth still blamed other people for his condition.

Although an extreme example, Gareth's approach to his health is something I sadly see in less severe forms time and time again. Essentially, Gareth's story is one of denial; from failing to document accurately what he ate to refusing to take the medication he was prescribed. It was obvious from the start that Gareth ate more than he wrote down, but this was his way of fighting back against a system that he either didn't trust or did not believe in. For whatever reason, Garath could not, or would not, accept that his poor lifestyle choices were contributing to his decline in health. His reluctance to engage with the medical therapies and lifestyle advice suggested highlighted Gareth's lack of acceptance of his condition, and even after he was permanently disabled by the damage done to his heart, he still blamed others for his decline in health.

As a doctor, it is important to remember that although we might prescribe medicines, perform operations and advise or educate on a variety of health matters, ultimately it is down to the individual patient to act on our recommendations. Some people might choose to disregard the medical advice given to them, which can be particularly hard to accept when, as doctors, we are trained to do the best for our patients. But no matter how hard we try, medicine can never be a substitute for taking responsibility for our own health.

CHAPTER 2

Fitness, Wellness and Cardiovascular Health

A s our jobs and lifestyles have made us more sedentary, the importance of physical fitness is now more relevant than ever before. But it is not just fitness that has become more popular in today's society. We are now constantly bombarded by adverts, recommendations and celebrities who, in addition to fitness, promote a way of life that we are told we should want to aspire to. With that expectation comes specific diets, exercise regimes, supplements and ideals for the way we are supposed to look. When we see the cover of male health or fitness magazines they are always depicting a muscular and shredded topless man, who appears joyful and elated with his Adonis-like physique. But what is it that actually draws us to these publications, and why do so many fitness apps and workout programmes even exist?

The pressures to look good

When it comes to male wellness, the decision to purchase a magazine, app or book usually comes down to either vanity, the desire to get lighter, fitter or healthier, or a combination of these. When it comes to vanity, Hollywood and the media have been instrumental in promoting the image of what it believes the ideal man should look like. It is now routine for high-profile celebrities to undergo months of gruelling fitness and diet regimes to look good for their films, and with the greater acceptance of the aesthetics of bodybuilding, we now spend more time than ever before trying to get big biceps and six packs – all in an attempt to match the image of what we feel we should look like. A good example of this is Hugh Jackman who starred in the X-Men Hollywood films playing the role of Wolverine. In 2000, when the first film was released, Jackman was 32 years old, he was athletic and had clearly worked out for the role. In 2017, Jackman played the same character in the film *Logan*, but despite being 17 years older, he was considerably more well built than in previous films. Jackman is open about the amount of training and effort that was required to achieve this level of physical fitness, and it is not something that would be sustainable in the long term. Nevertheless, it is a particularly good example of how the same character, played by the same actor 17 years apart, has had to change his on-screen appearance based on the expectations of the modern male body image.

Even compared with when I started going to the gym, now over 20 years ago, the sheer volume of people that now lift weights is incredible, and fitness and bodybuilding have become an accepted part of mainstream culture. Up until the last few years, gyms were seen as places to focus on getting better at your primary sport or the home of odd dysmorphic bodybuilders; however, as the concept of the ideal male body has been distorted and pushed upon us through TV and social media, more than ever, teenagers and young men are feeling the pressure to obtain the perfect physique. There has also been a steep rise in the use of anabolic steroids in an attempt to try to reach unobtainable goals or shortcut many years of work. Not only does this carry with it the risk of long-term physical damage but it is also directly associated with an increased incidence of mental-health problems. Sadly, the pressure to look a certain way can have marked negative effects on the psychological well-being of many younger men, and recently I have seen many more cases of male body dysmorphia presenting to my clinic. These are fit and healthy young men who believe that because they are not able to achieve the superhuman physiques of pro-bodybuilders or actors they see on screen, they must have low testosterone. In reality, and in virtually all cases, this is a delusional belief about how we see ourselves. It is similar to anorexia and results in the sufferer never being satisfied with what he sees in the mirror. Unsurprisingly, this can have very negative long-term effects on mental wellness and the ability to accept who we are as we age.

The good side of vanity

Vanity, however, and the aspiration to look like the man on the front cover of a magazine, is not necessarily a bad thing. Vanity helps us to lose weight, it makes us work harder, take pride in our appearance and strive to get good grades or excel in sports. In essence, vanity can be the positive consequence of our insecurities, and it keeps us motivated. Of course, in the extreme, vanity can be a highly negative aspect of our personalities. The number of women and men in my gym who film their training so that it can be posted on social media in the desperate hope of another virtual thumbs up, is simply maddening. But, in essence, the desire to self-improve, take pride in our appearance and be the best version of ourselves we can, is not a bad thing.

Another reason we take an interest in health and wellness media is to get better at a specific sport we play or enjoy. Following a particular sports personality or team is not only fun but it can also provide inspiration and guidance on how to improve performance. The majority of people who play a sport regularly can usually name at least a few of the top athletes in that field and are also likely to be broadly aware of their training regime. There is no doubt that whatever physical activity we participate in, we are likely to benefit from the experience offered by those at the top.

The final reason people take an interest in health and

fitness media is to help educate them on getting fitter. This might be because they noticed changes in the way they look, or the desire to achieve a specific target, such as the 'Couch to 5k'. Of course, there is some crossover with vanity, but many people take up a sport or physical activity in an effort to simply improve their overall health, athletic performance or sense of well-being.

Fitness for health rather than appearance

In contrast to these common motives to exercise, it is almost unheard of for someone to enter into a sport or exercise regime because they specifically want to reduce their blood pressure or cholesterol without being told to do so by a health professional. Primary disease prevention is far from a common reason people join a gym. But as men, if we knew how influential exercise was in reducing our heart disease and stroke risk, even without knowing our cholesterol or blood pressure, it is likely that more of us might be convinced to get fit.

In 2016, the World Health Organization (WHO) recorded heart disease and stroke as the world's biggest killers, accounting for a combined 15.2 million deaths worldwide.[1] In general, men develop the conditions that lead to heart disease (specifically high blood pressure, cholesterol and diabetes) at a younger age than women, and they also have a higher chance of developing coronary heart damage. Even though women are more likely to suffer a stroke than men, this is seen more in later life only. Overall, deaths from strokes and heart disease are highest in middle-aged men, and this statistic persists for most of our lives.

Whereas we might worry about the size of our biceps, or if our 5k run is fast enough, perhaps we also need to think more actively about what is actually happening inside our bodies and whether we are doing everything we can to prepare ourselves for the future?

What is cardiovascular disease?

We tend to think of cardiovascular disease (CVD) as referring to a heart attack. But CVD is a general term used to describe a range of conditions that affect the heart or blood vessels. CVD is a process by which multiple conditions, such as high blood pressure, high cholesterol, and type-2 diabetes, contribute to a gradual narrowing of the arteries within the body. As the arteries are damaged, they build up layers of fatty deposits that make the blood flow increasingly difficult (atherosclerosis). This eventually results in a clot and the subsequent loss of blood supply to whichever organ that artery was supplying. When this process occurs in the heart, this is a heart attack and, similarly, when this happens in the brain, the result is a stroke; however, since arteries provide the blood supply to every organ in the body, CVD can affect anywhere, from the legs, penis, kidneys and even our eyes. The arteries in the penis are in fact so similar to those in the heart that there is a general rule in medicine that once you develop erectile dysfunction due to CVD there will be three-year window where you are almost certain to suffer a heart attack.

The effect of cardiovascular disease on the
arteries that supply the heart

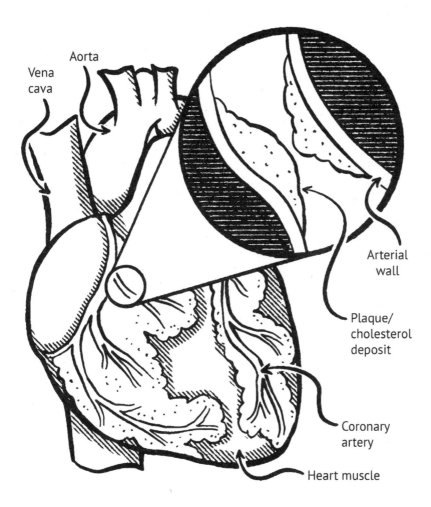

Vena cava

Aorta

Arterial wall

Plaque/ cholesterol deposit

Coronary artery

Heart muscle

The history of heart disease

Throughout history the recording and documentation of heart attacks has been, until relatively recently, focused almost exclusively on men. Even taking into account that

historically medicine and literature were highly male cen-
tred, the development of chest pain and heart attacks has
always been a predominately male problem.

It is likely that to some extent heart disease has been
present in men for thousands of years. In 2009 the *Journal
of the American Medical Association* presented their study
of a 3,500-year-old Egyptian mummy who was scanned
and found to have heart disease, specifically atherosclerosis,
which, as we have seen, is the process of narrowed arteries
that leads to a heart attack. Interestingly, this was not a
unique finding. Atherosclerosis was present in the arteries
of several mummified bodies from more than 3,500 years
ago. This raises the question as to whether our modern lifestyle is really the leading cause of heart disease, or is there
something deeper in our male DNA?

It is not entirely clear when the link between atherosclerosis
and heart attacks was made, but most accounts tend to date
back to the 18th century; for example, Friedrich Hoffmann
(1660–1742), chief professor of medicine at the University of
Halle in Germany, documented that heart disease was related
to a 'reduced passage of the blood within the coronary arteries'.[2] Only a few years later, London's John Hunter, a highly
respected surgeon, successfully documented his own episodes
of worsening chest pain and actually died storming out of a
board meeting at St George's Hospital in 1793.[3] His post-
mortem found that he had indeed died from heart disease.

It wasn't until the early 20th century that the link was
made between cardiac chest pain (known as angina) and a
narrowing of the coronary arteries. In addition, it wasn't
until much later that century that specific treatments for

heart attacks became available. Even in the limited time I have been a doctor, treatments have progressed so rapidly that when I started in medicine we used to give heart-attack patients a massive dose of an intravenous clot-busting drug, which we hoped would dissolve the blockage before too much damage was done to their heart. The problem with this medication was that not only did it take time to work, which is especially important in a condition where for every minute the artery remains blocked further damage is being done to the heart muscle, but it also massively increased the risk of bleeding elsewhere in the body.

The changes in the way we now treat heart attacks have been so successful that we have effectively made many cardio-thoracic surgeons redundant. Previously, despite the use of clot-dissolving medications, significant numbers of patients who suffered heart attacks would still have to undergo open-heart surgery to transplant a blood vessel from one part of their body (usually the leg or arm) and literally plumb it into the heart to replace the blocked and damaged vessel which, for whatever reason, could not be successfully treated with intravenous medicine.

Now confirmed heart-attack patients go straight to the cardiologist's 'cath lab' where, under specialist guidance, a small wire is inserted up through the side of the pelvis and passed up into the heart, then a little balloon or stent is used to open the artery again. Because heart attacks can now be managed so quickly and effectively with minimal cutting or risk to the patient, and under a local anaesthetic, the need for a cardio-thoracic surgeon to open up the chest and plumb in new vessels has all but disappeared.

Why are men more likely to suffer a heart attack than women?

We still don't know exactly why men are more susceptible to heart attacks than women. Perhaps unsurprisingly, therefore, we find that there are many different possibilities when looking into the reasons why men have more cardiovascular problems than women. Broadly, however, these reasons can be separated into those things we can alter, such as lifestyle factors or blood pressure, and those we cannot, such as hormones and genes.

One common theory as to why CVD rates are higher in men is the fact that the raised levels of oestrogen in women in some way protects them against heart disease. Evidence suggests, however, that even after menopause (when oestrogen levels in women drop to virtually zero) the risk of women suffering from a heart attack increases only slightly. Another theory suggests that because men are more likely to present to their doctor with the classic symptoms of heart-attack pain, they are therefore more commonly diagnosed.

What to look out for

The typical symptoms of a heart attack include:

- Severe, crushing chest pain down the left side that can also radiate out to the left arm and/or neck
- Shortness of breath

- Racing heart
- Nausea
- Feeling dizzy or near fainting

There has been some evidence to suggest that women present to hospital later with fewer of the classic symptoms listed in the box above and often express less pain. As a result, the suggestion is that more heart attacks in women are missed; however, in 2018 this theory was contested, and it has now been suggested that the majority of both women and men suffer the symptoms of having a heart attack in the same way.[4]

There is no doubt that developments in medicine and technology have significantly improved the survival rates for both sexes in terms of CVD, with the numbers of deaths relating to heart attacks and strokes declining considerably in the last 30 years. But despite this, the numbers of men dying from heart disease remains consistently higher than women until they both reach old age. Furthermore, this statistic remains true across a range of economically, socially and culturally diverse countries.[5]

Therefore, if it is not women's hormones that protect them from CVD, or the way we diagnose chest pain, or even the fact that we can save more people than ever before, why do men still suffer with heart disease and its complications more frequently than women? In reality, it is not that complicated. There are some major risk factors that are largely attributable to simply being male that put us at an increased risk of CVD, many of which we can do something about.

Low testosterone

There are some suggestions that, compared with women, the higher levels of testosterone produced in men could directly result in an increased risk of CVD, but this is simply not true. Normal levels of testosterone do not increase the chances of cardiovascular damage. In fact, it is now accepted that *low* levels of testosterone in men are directly linked to an *increased* risk of heart disease and type-2 diabetes. Interestingly, CVD risk also rises in men who abuse anabolic steroids and who take their testosterone levels above the normal physiological range. Therefore, the best way to think about testosterone levels in terms of CVD risk is to think of it as a bell-shaped curve: too low and you increase your chances of high blood pressure, high cholesterol and obesity; too high, and it also increases the risk of high blood pressure and the production of too many red blood cells. Either way, both result it an increased risk of blood getting stuck in the arteries and causing a blockage.

Stress

We all get stressed. When this is short-lived, it is a normal physiological process and has no long-term adverse effects on our health. But the same cannot be said for men who suffer with persistent stress, anger or chronic anxiety. Prolonged stress disorders result in a rise in blood pressure and the release of stress hormones, both of which can lead to a restriction in blood flow to the heart and other vital organs. There have even been recent studies that have suggested that during acutely stressful events the brain actively releases specific types of white cells that increase levels of inflammation in the arteries and actually reduce their blood flow.[6] It is not unheard of for a man to be in the throes of a violent outburst, only for this to bring the onset of a heart attack.

The shapes of our bodies

In general, women have higher percentages of body fat than men, typically 25 per cent for women at a healthy weight compared with 15 per cent for men. This is partly owing to the fact that production of female hormones such as oestrogen makes it easier to convert food into fat. We all know that having more fat is bad for us, so if women have around 10 per cent more body fat than men, shouldn't this contribute to an increase in CVD? As with much else in medicine, things are not that simple. In reality, it is not just the total volume of excess fat we carry that increases our risk of CVD but where this excess fat sits. The phrase 'a moment on the lips, a lifetime on the hips', is really only applicable to the way women deposit excess fat, as for men it is more a case of 'food that tastes yummy, ends up on your tummy'. Women are considered to be 'pear shaped', that is, excess fat tends to get stored on the hips and thighs (and in the breast tissue), whereas men tend to be more 'apple shaped', with fat being distributed largely around the midsection.

In addition to where it is stored, women's excess fat tends to be deposited more superficially (often resulting in the classic cellulite appearance). But although potentially cosmetically distressing, this superficial fat has little effect

Typical fat distribution in men and women

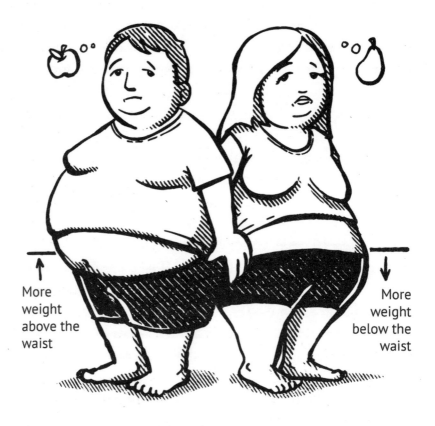

More
weight
above the
waist

More
weight
below the
waist

on the internal organs and arteries. In contrast, men's fat is stored around their midsection (and is known as visceral fat). It is much more harmful and has multiple adverse effects on the body. Visceral fat surrounds vital organs such as the liver, intestines and heart. This fat is poorly stored, and tends to get released into the arteries and surrounding tissues. In addition, visceral fat is particularly harmful to our hormone pathways, reducing testosterone, making us resistant to insulin and increasing oestrogen levels. Visceral fat has even been linked to the release of specific pro-inflammatory immune proteins that can result in damage to various organs. Overall, visceral fat is considered to be so significant as a potential contributor towards CVD that waistline measurement is sometimes more important than overall body weight. NHS guidelines advise that regardless of height or body mass index (BMI), you should try to lose weight if your waist is more than 94cm (37in) for a man, and more than 80cm (31½in) for a woman.

Blood pressure

High blood pressure increases our risk of CVD by literally increasing the pressure in the circulatory system. If the pressure stays high for long enough, eventually it will start to cause damage to the lining of the arteries, which allows cholesterol to stick and the narrowing process to begin. It appears that oestrogen in women is protective in keeping blood pressure down, and their levels quickly rise to match male levels after menopause. Men's arteries tend to be more sensitive to the effects of salt in their diet, as well as being more reactive to life pressures, hence the reason why our blood pressure goes up more than women's when we are stressed. The reason stress results in high blood pressure is because of a series of physiological responses that involve adrenaline release, increased heart rate and constriction of the arteries. Even at a relatively young age, this makes men's arteries more susceptible to the effects of poor lifestyle choices, and this small but cumulative damage can go on to lead to significant problems later on in life.

Cholesterol

We spend so much time talking about reducing our cholesterol, or making sure that we don't eat too many 'bad fats', that our understanding of what cholesterol really is has been distorted and it is now perceived as something entirely negative. Cholesterol is a waxy, fat-like substance that is produced in our liver and also found in some foods. It is present in most cells in our bodies and, despite what we might hear, we need it to survive. Cholesterol forms part of the outer layer of cell membranes and is especially important for brain, nerve and skin function. It is required to make vitamin D and many hormones (including testosterone), and it is also used to produce bile, which helps to digest our food.

There are several types of cholesterol, but the two we most commonly hear about are HDL (high-density lipoprotein), and LDL (low-density lipoprotein). LDL cholesterol has been dubbed 'bad' because having too much in the blood can lead to an increase in CVD. The main role of LDL is to deliver cholesterol to the cells that need it, but when there is more LDL in our bodies than is required, it builds up and can stick to our arteries, leading to narrowing of the vessels and subsequent cardiovascular disease. In contrast, HDL is the 'good' cholesterol because it has lots of protein in it, and its main job is to take cholesterol away from the blood and put it in the liver where it can be metabolised and then removed from the body.

Women naturally have higher levels of the good HDL cholesterol levels than men. Once again, this is due to the protective effects of female hormones, which disappear after menopause as cholesterol levels in men and women equalise.

The biggest problem with cholesterol is that although we need it to survive, we don't need very much. From an evolutionary perspective, historically, high-quality food, in particular fat, was a rarity in our diets so our brains evolved to favour those foods with a high fat content. In a modern Western diet, however, fat is so readily incorporated into our daily menu that it is extremely hard for us to avoid eating more than we need.

Lifestyle and behaviour

The traditional, stereotypical narrative that men go out to work while women look after the home has lessened in the 21st century, but there is still a cultural pressure that exists for many men in terms of the way they work and are expected to socialise. A large proportion of men still work long hours, spend more time commuting than women and are expected to participate in the 'lad' culture of drinking and socialising. The consequence of this is a cocktail of socio-economic pressures that adds further risk to male health.

The UK has a reputation as being a nation of heavy drinkers. Whether this is drinking wine at home with our partner or through enjoying a few beers with our friends in the pub, there is no doubt that as a population we are unique in our high levels of alcohol consumption. The current UK guidelines on alcohol consumption advise no more than 14 units a week for women and men. This is equivalent to drinking 6 pints of beer or 7 medium-sized glasses of wine. In 2017, in England, 24 per cent of men said that their average weekly alcohol consumption was more than the recommended amount, compared with only 11 per cent of women.[7] This is not to suggest that women do not play their part in contributing to binge drinking, alcoholism and liver disease, but it is just that the numbers are higher in men and their underlying risk factors are already greater.

In the long term, heavy drinking can lead to an increase in CVD via several different mechanisms, including a rise in blood pressure, a reduction in testosterone levels, increased consumption of calories resulting in obesity and even causing a direct stress on the heart muscle. The long-peddled notion that a glass of wine a day could actually be beneficial for us in terms of heart health is not based on good science. Many of the early studies looked at complete abstinence compared with a moderate or minimal alcohol intake, but it is now understood that many of the participants who did not drink at all did so because of pre-existing health reasons, which increased their overall risk of CVD. In more recent studies, it has become apparent that people who consume a moderate amount of alcohol (rather than the extreme of too little or too much) also tend to be more well educated, exercise more and eat healthier. These confounding factors mean that it is extremely difficult to determine what are the true effects of alcohol on heart disease and stroke risk. Sadly, the current consensus is that there are no proven cardiac benefits to drinking alcohol.

My clinic is populated with large numbers of men who set off for work before sunrise, drive hundreds of miles a week and get home after dark. Their lunch is a petrol-station sandwich, and their main way to unwind is through alcohol. Because their jobs are all-consuming, it can make changes in behaviour extremely difficult.

Reducing the risk of cardiovascular disease

What can really be done to keep you healthy and reduce your risk of cardiovascular disease? At first glance, it seems that there are so many factors that contribute to the development of CVD in men that it is a futile endeavour to try to stop this juggernaut of disease heading towards us. Oddly, in some respects you would be right, and the first thing to remember when trying to optimise your health is that we cannot alter our genes. As we have already established, simply being male increases your chances of CVD – and just as we can't stop getting older, we can't stop being male. These unalterable aspects of ourselves are known as 'irreversible risk factors' and need to be discounted before we go any further. In contrast, the list of 'modifiable risk factors', or things that we *can* change about our health, is still significant, and we can make major improvements to our general well-being and risk of illness by addressing them.

Maintain a healthy weight

Other than drugs (such as smoking or alcohol), diet is the number-one modifiable risk factor for heart disease and cardiovascular health in men. We are told time and time again, that not only what we eat, but also how much we eat, play a critical role in keeping us healthy.

One of the biggest challenges we face in the battle to eat well is the disparity between what we think we are eating and what we actually consume. Recently, the British Social Attitudes Survey looked at people's perceptions and understanding of obesity.[8] Nearly three-quarters of those who took the survey knew that most people who are overweight are like this because they eat too much. Nearly 90 per cent of those who replied also agreed that eating a healthier diet and doing more physical activity are both crucial in helping someone to lose weight. But when the Office for National Statistics published their paper about perceptions of food, they found that typically men underestimated what they consume by 1,000 calories a day.[9] But this is not a revelation, and it is something I have witnessed on many occasions in my own clinic. Most of the time this underestimation of calorie intake is not a deliberate attempt to deceive the doctor, but it is an unconscious delusion about how much we actually ingest. Our brain does not want us to appear as slobs, so it tends to miscalculate the amount of food that we actually eat.

Accepting the fact that we do indeed tend to eat more than we need, it is essential that if we are going to lose weight we do it through an evidence-based and logical approach. With so many companies and products touting the best or newest way to get slim, it can be a daunting task to decide what is legitimate and what is just magic beans.

In practice, weight loss is not that complicated, and the overall principle is straightforward: ingest fewer calories than you expend and over a given period of time, your body weight will drop. It really is that simple, but there are clear genetic differences in the way that we are built, how we store fat and how we metabolise our food. It can be incredibly disheartening for someone who has made great efforts with their diet and exercise to see minimal progress while their friend, who eats junk food all day and does no exercise, remains thin. It is important to accept that we are different, and while the principle of eat less, move more, applies to everybody, the way this message is delivered and applied has to vary from person to person to be effective. Clearly, the health and wellness industry would not be as lucrative as it is if their message to everyone was just to eat less food. It is actually our individuality that allows this industry to thrive, focusing on our personal preferences for ways of eating, types of food we favour or ways to exercise and play sport.

An added difficulty in achieving what should be a simple 'less in' process is made harder because our lives and bodies want us to do the opposite. Genetically, we crave high-sugar and high-fat foods, our lifestyles are rarely conducive to exercising and napping when we want, and our social structures mean that we tend to eat meals and drink alcohol when we meet friends. The other big problem is that dieting is just unpleasant. No one likes to feel the pain of hunger, snack on celery, meet friends for a Diet Coke or choose a rice cake over chocolate cake. As a result, there is a role for the health and fitness industry to sell us products that help us to achieve our goal in a way that suits our individual lifestyle, gives us structure and minimises the unpleasant aspects of the dieting process. The problem comes because so many companies have observed the difficulty we suffer when trying to lose weight, and so they capitalise on a desperate market by offering get-thin-quick pills or diets, the vast majority of which do nothing. With that in mind, the following section reviews some of the most popular current diet plans and looks at the evidence to show whether they are easy to follow and safe, and whether they actually work.

The ketogenic (keto) diet

Keto diets have actually been around for nearly one hundred years and were originally used in the treatment of epilepsy in the 1920s and 1930s. Although quite successful in treating this illness, the introduction of anticonvulsant medication made the diet largely redundant, with only a very small proportion of epilepsy patients still using it. In the last 15 years, however, keto diets have seen an explosion in popularity, not in the treatment of neurological illnesses but as a way to lose weight or potentially live a healthier lifestyle. But what does the keto diet actually mean?

Keto diets refer to an umbrella term for any diet that places a greater emphasis on us obtaining our calories by eating protein and fat rather than carbohydrates. Examples of keto diets include the Paleo and the Atkins diet, both of which are discussed in more detail later on. But it is important to differentiate between what is a low-carbohydrate diet (often termed keto) and a true ketogenic diet, which has profoundly different effects on the body.

Most keto diets are actually low-carb diets, with ingested carbohydrates representing about 10–30 per cent of the daily calories consumed compared with a conventional Western diet, which is usually 45–60 per cent carbohydrate.

In general, low-carb diets can be healthy; they are good at helping us to lose weight and are often promoted in the treatment, and even reversal, of some forms of type-2 diabetes.

In true ketogenic diets, however, the percentage of daily carbohydrate consumed is actually far less than a conventional low-carb diet, with the aim being to consume as little carbohydrate as possible. In doing so, the dieter substitutes their calorie requirements with protein and fat. This results in a metabolic shift that causes the liver to produce ketones from fat, which are then used for energy rather than carbohydrates being converted to simple sugars. This process of ketosis can be achieved only by consuming fewer than 50 grams of carbs per day (bearing in mind a single banana has around 27 grams of carbohydrate) while keeping protein intake moderate and drastically increasing the daily intake of fat.

Obviously, by entering into this state of fat-burning ketosis, it can induce significant weight loss, as the fat we are eating is being primarily used as metabolic fuel rather than being stored as body fat. But one of the biggest misconceptions in ketogenic diets is that eating high levels of protein is also beneficial. In true ketogenic diets, the only way to reach a ketotic state, whereby we use fat as our primary fuel instead of glucose, is to have no other additional energy sources, and this includes protein. As such, a keto diet that is high in fat and protein is not truly ketogenic at all.

Even if the idea of eating fat for the majority of all your meals and snacks every day was not unpalatable enough, there are obvious safety implications in following this sort of diet in the long term. We know that a ketogenic diet reduces seizures in some epileptic children, but there is no evidence to support suggestions that the diet might also offer some protection against other neurological conditions such as Parkinson's disease or Alzheimer's disease. In addition, there have been questions raised about the effects that such a high-fat diet could have on levels of cholesterol in our bodies and on the heart and cardiovascular system, and whether it might adversely affect our risk of CVD. Ketogenic diets also lead to other problems that are associated with low vegetable and fruit consumption, such as constipation and vitamin deficiencies. But what about other, less severe, keto diets?

The Paleo diet

A Paleo diet is based on foods similar to those early man might have been eating during the Palaeolithic era, from the emergence of early Stone Age man around 3 million years ago, until approximately 10,000 years ago and the start of the first agricultural era. As such, it limits food choices to mainly protein sources, with some fruit and vegetables, and few, if any, complex carbohydrates. The rationale behind the Paleo diet is that the human body is genetically mismatched to our modern ways of eating, and that the agricultural revolution changed the way we consume food, resulting in what is known as the discordance hypothesis where what we are encouraged to consume by our society and culture does not match what we have evolved to require. In general, Paleo diets consist of fruit, vegetables, nuts, seeds, meat – especially grass-fed animals – fish and oils.

The Paleo diet fits under the umbrella term of keto

because it excludes whole grains, dairy and legumes (peas, beans and pulses), and relies on a higher intake of protein and fat. It is not ketogenic, but it can aid weight loss due to a general reduction in carbohydrate consumption. One of the main problems with the Paleo diet is that by excluding specific foods it can remove essential sources of fibre, calcium, vitamins and other nutrients. There is also much debate about just how accurate the Paleo diet really is in matching what Palaeolithic man would have eaten.

The Atkins diet

Dr Robert Atkins was an American cardiologist who attempted to apply the principles of the low-carb/keto diet to help improve his own weight issues. In 1972 the Atkins diet was published, which is effectively similar to a ketogenic diet. It consists of virtually no carbohydrates for the first two weeks, followed by the gradual introduction of small amounts of carbohydrate to make the diet more tolerable. Unlike a true ketogenic diet, there is less restriction on protein intake, but a high fat intake is encouraged. As carbohydrates are reintroduced, the dieter is meant to assess how much carbohydrate is required to keep their weight stable. Dieters are also actively encouraged to exercise.

As with true ketogenic diets, there are no studies that have looked at the safety or long-term effects of the Paleo or Atkins diet on our bodies. It is relatively safe to say that diets low in carbohydrates are beneficial in helping us to reduce weight by providing an overall reduction in calorie consumption. But these diets are all restrictive, and they substitute carbohydrates with an increased intake of fat and, to a lesser extent, protein. Concerns should be raised about any diet that excludes any specific food group, and we just do not know what the long-term effects of a high-fat diet, in particular one that is high in saturated fat, might have on our cardiovascular health. Although the link between high keto diets and CVD risk might not be as obvious as first predicted, currently we just do not know for sure. When advising patients on nutrition, the difficulty health professionals face is trying to juggle what is known to be effective in the short term at reducing the risk of obesity-related disease, with what evidence we have about the effects of specific diets on our long-term health. For now, the debate continues.

> ### Myth buster: true or false?
>
> Myth: a quick detox diet will help me to lose weight and feel better.
>
> *False.* There is no such thing as a detox. You have a liver and kidneys that process and remove waste products from your body better than anything you can eat, drink or rub on. When you detox you might feel better if you have eaten more healthily during that detox period, but never get tricked into thinking that a product will in some way be more effective than your own body.

Intermittent fasting

The principal difference between intermittent fasting and most other forms of diet is that it restricts *when* you can eat, not *what* you can eat. Much like a lot of other health and wellness products, the concept of intermittent fasting has been around for many years. From an evolutionary perspective, we would not continually graze, and often we would only eat every few days, based on the availability of food. Gradually over time, our lives have become more sedentary, obtaining the food we need requires less and less physical effort and we are able to access food at any time of the day or night.

Intermittent fasting works by setting a predetermined time each day that food can be consumed. This restricts the total time we are able to eat in a 24-hour period and consequently reduces our total calorie intake. In addition, if we go long enough without food, our sugar stores are used up and we start using fat as our primary energy source. This is very similar to the ketosis observed in ketogenic diets, but it works by metabolising our existing fat stores rather than trying to convert the additional fat that we eat.

There are several different types of intermittent fasting, including alternate-day fasting, daily time-restricted feeding and periodic fasting, the most famous of which is the 5:2 diet. Although the diet already existed, it was made popular by Michael Mosley in 2012 following a BBC documentary on the topic. The process itself is relatively simple and involves eating normally for five days of the week and having two days where calories are restricted to 500–600 per day. On the low-calorie days, water and other zero-calorie beverages such as black coffee and tea are permitted. And during the five days of normal eating, this means consuming a healthy balanced diet; it should not be considered a free pass to eat whatever we want as a treat for fasting the day before.

In general, the success and health benefits of intermittent fasting seem very positive. In the short term, users do develop some irritability and tiredness on the days when they fast, but most people seem to get to used to this and some also notice that over time, even on days when they can eat normally, their desire to consume large meals decreases. In the medium term, intermittent fasting helps to reduce body weight, improves insulin sensitivity and release, which improves blood sugar levels, and it can improve health conditions such as type-2 diabetes.

In the long term, however, the health benefits or risks for intermittent fasting are not as well established, and, just like keto diets, we just don't know the long-term health implications of severely restricting food intake over decades.

The Dukan diet

Invented by Dr Pierre Dukan in the 1970s, the Dukan diet is a high-protein, low-carbohydrate diet that essentially has four phases and starts with a virtually protein-only diet for one week. The main difference between this and the Paleo or Atkins diets is that in the first phase of the Dukan plan vegetables are prohibited and fat intake is significantly restricted. The next three phases of the plan see a gradual reintroduction of some fruit, vegetables and carbs, and eventually all foods. The main principle of the diet is to stick to low-fat, low-salt and high-protein foods, and there are no restrictions on how much you can eat during the first two weeks.

The downside with the diet is that it is hard to sustain in the long term. The extreme reduction in carbohydrates in the first week can cause marked side effects of dizziness, fatigue, irritability and concentration problems owing to the sudden lack of quick and usable carbohydrate energy. It is also hard to maintain such a high protein intake over the long term and has largely been advocated as a quick way to lose weight but not something that most people will adhere to as a permanent lifestyle adaptation.

The alkaline diet

Dating back as far as the early 20th century, the alkaline diet is based on the idea that by altering the pH (acidity or alkalinity) of our bodies we can improve or worsen our overall health. Advocates of the alkaline diet believe that certain foods can affect our blood pH and that by increasing the pH, or making us less acidic, this can treat or prevent disease. High acidity has been blamed on increased body fat, arthritis, osteoporosis, tiredness, and kidney and liver disorders.

There is no credible data to support any of this. The diet involves reducing supposedly acid-producing foods such as meat, wheat, sugar, dairy products, caffeine, alcohol and processed foods. In contrast, foods that are supposed to be alkaline include fruit and vegetables.

It is easy to see how following the diet would result in some health benefits and very likely also cause weight loss, but even at a basic level the science behind it makes no sense. Normal blood pH is 7.40 and even small variations in this (such as a pH of less than 7.35) can make us extremely sick. The body is highly efficient at maintaining a constant pH, and it does so through the actions of the lungs and kidneys. The carbon dioxide we breathe out is very slightly acidic, and our brains can very simply increase or decrease our pH at a minute level just by taking more breaths. The kidneys can excrete acid or alkaline substances into the blood over a slower period, but this is also driven centrally by the actions of the brain. You can eat anything you want, and it will not alter your blood pH. More importantly, there is no scientific basis for any aspect of this diet, and it is therefore best avoided.

Weight Watchers, Slim Fast, Slimming World

Even though Weight Watchers, Slim Fast and Slimming World are all individual diet plans, I have grouped them together because, unlike keto or intermittent fasting, which are dietary concepts, these are all commercial products in themselves and require the dieter to sign up to a plan or product. These brands are all calorie-control diets and work by either replacing meals, swapping high-calorie foods for low-calorie ones, or assigning points to foods based on their calorie count. Although there are differences in the way the programmes are run, they all actively encourage the intake of fruit and vegetables, and no foods are really banned.

The success of diet plans like these often rely on the user following, and paying for, the advice and continued support the programme or product offers; for example, with Slim Fast the user has to buy meal replacement drinks to adhere to the diet plan, and with Weight Watchers, users are encouraged to attend group meetings or sign up to online programmes, products and support. These diets, in particular Weight Watchers and Slimming World, can offer a good basis for a healthy diet, and can be a useful introduction into long-term healthy eating. (I would not, however, advocate the long-term use of meal replacements instead of actual food.)

The Mediterranean diet

There are many other diets available that I have not included in this chapter, but those listed above provide a summary of the most common principles of different weight-loss plans. I have also included the Mediterranean diet, not because it is promoted as a way to lose weight but because it is often held as an ideal of how we should be eating.

The Mediterranean diet varies by country and region, of course, so it has a range of definitions. In the UK, the traditional Mediterranean diet has been adapted to illustrate a simple and healthy way of eating that is essentially high in vegetables, fruits, legumes (peas, beans and lentils), nuts, beans, cereals, grains and fish, as well as unsaturated fats such as olive oil. It does not exclude any food group, but has a lower intake of meat and dairy foods than can be found in some Mediterranean countries. In fact, the Mediterranean diet is considered so beneficial that the World Health Organization has listed it as a healthy and sustainable dietary pattern.

Eating the Mediterranean way

The key elements of the Mediterranean diet are:

- Eat more fruit and vegetables. Aim for seven to ten servings a day.
- Don't avoid carbohydrates, but switch to whole-grain bread, cereal and pasta.
- Use healthy fats. Use olive oil as a replacement for butter when cooking. Avoid unsaturated fats where possible.
- Eat more seafood, at least twice a week. Ideally, this should be oily fish such as tuna, salmon, trout, mackerel and sardines.
- Keep red meat to a minimum. If you eat meat, make sure it is not processed and try to stick to lean meats.
- Enjoy some dairy. Dairy still provides protein, calcium and various vitamins. Eaten in moderation, it does not have to be avoided.

I am firm believer that there are no quick results when it comes to weight loss and health. If you wish to eat more healthily, the concept of the Mediterranean diet is good because it contains all the food groups in appropriate amounts. Also, you don't have to buy a product to adhere to the diet. The downside is that it may not be prescriptive enough for some people who need more specific advice on how to reduce total calorie intake or where they can improve aspects of their diet.

Even as a type-1 diabetic myself, I am not keen on very low-carbohydrate diets. We require carbs to give us energy, and they are an essential fuel for exercise and sporting activity, as well as for our brains, which rely on carbohydrates as its primary energy source. Intermittent fasting can be a great way to lose weight if done safely, but without additional guidance it teaches us to eat less but not necessarily healthier. I would also always steer clear of any diet that is restrictive and advocates complete abstinence of one or multiple types of food. Overall, if you are wishing to lose weight, intermittent fasting, reduced-carb diets, or calorie-counting programmes are probably fine in the short term. (Obviously, though, this should be taken in the context of your underlying health, and if in doubt, please speak to your doctor before commencing a diet plan that you are not sure about.) In the long run, we should be aiming to adhere to a more Mediterranean-style way of eating, but this can be difficult when everything around us is still tempting us to eat chocolate and crisps.

Take exercise

When it comes to simple weight loss, exercise is less important than diet. This is because even vigorous exercise uses only a fraction of our total calorie intake; for example, it takes around 22 minutes of running to burn off a chocolate bar, equivalent to less than one-tenth of a man's daily calorie intake. But this does not mean that exercise is not as important as what we eat, it just means that its benefits come from helping to maintain our weight once we have lost excess fat, as well as providing a broader range of health benefits that significantly contribute to reducing the risk of CVD.

At a basic level, physical activity provides increased blood flow to muscles. Locally, this promotes growth of the muscles used, and it can also improve bone density and blood vessel stimulation. Over time, exercise can even improve the blood flow to organs affected by atherosclerosis (blocked arteries) and can actually undo some of the harmful effects of CVD. In addition to this, exercise stimulates testosterone release, increases our levels of HDL cholesterol and reduces blood pressure. Physical activity has even been shown to reduce our risk of cancer and type-2 diabetes. From a mental-health perspective, exercise releases endorphins that make us feel good, it reduces depression and anxiety, helps us to sleep, gives us more energy, and it can even reduce the progression of dementia.

How, then, do we know which type of exercise is best? Exercise can be split into three basic groups: aerobic (cardiovascular fitness); strength training and weights; and flexibility and balance. In terms of which is best, there is no single ideal form of activity. Each type of exercise has its own benefits, and often what we choose to do is based on our health needs, individual goals and ultimately what we enjoy. Most importantly, whatever we choose, it has to be something sustainable.

Aerobic
Aerobic exercise is essentially any type of continuous activity that works your heart, lungs and muscles. It tends to be low impact, and examples include cycling, long-distance running and swimming. The main benefits of aerobic exercise are that it improves cardiovascular health and can reduce the risk of heart disease, type-2 diabetes and certain

cancers as well as improving mood and sleep. But aerobic exercise does not improve our flexibility, balance and coordination, nor does it increase muscle size or maintain bone density. Repeated, chronic aerobic activity, such as frequent, long-distance running or cycling can even cause suppression of testosterone production, not to mention the negative impact on joints through overall wear and tear.

Strength training

Previously referred to as anaerobic exercise, strength training focuses on building up or maintaining strength and size in our skeletal muscles, which is especially important as we age because we naturally lose muscle mass when we get older. An additional benefit of strength training is that it improves bone density by putting pressure on the skeleton, which helps to keep it healthy and reduce the risk of bone thinning and osteoporosis. This improved muscle mass and bone density can help in maintaining and improving daily activities and good posture, as well as preventing problems such as lower back pain. The downside with strength training, however, is that unless it is sufficiently intense, it might not stimulate the cardiovascular system enough to benefit heart health. In addition, poor technique, not warming up beforehand, and the use of overly heavy weights (known as 'ego lifting') can result in tendon and ligament injuries, and even complete muscle or tendon tears.

Flexibility training

A more static form of exercise, flexibility training promotes core strength, flexibility and good balance. As we age, our balance tends to decline, and the limited range of movements we perform in day-to-day life can shorten our muscle fibres and reduce flexibility. Although this type of exercise involves slowly stretching your muscles without jerking or bouncing them, it can still be extremely challenging. Examples include yoga, Pilates, and t'ai chi, all of which can improve core strength, balance and flexibility. The downside to flexibility training is that it might not be intense enough to provide the cardiovascular benefits of aerobic exercise, and it might not provide enough resistance to maintain the muscle and bone strength that would be achieved through strength training.

How much exercise do you need?

As well as deciding on the type of exercise that is best for you, the other question I am often asked is how much exercise do you need to do. There are various national and international guidelines on ideal exercise amounts, but at a very basic level any amount of aerobic exercise will be beneficial to your health. In terms of truly effective exercise for muscle growth and cardiovascular health, a good target to aim for is to do at least 150 minutes of moderate-intensity activity a week, or 75 minutes of vigorous-intensity activity a week. This should be split up into several sessions, and ideally I would aim to do something at least three or four times per week.

If you are trying to lose weight, it is important to remember that the exercise you perform needs to be in conjunction with a healthy diet. In terms of the ideal training regime, there is no single magic routine that will keep us supple, strong and fit. We need to tailor our exercise to our individual needs and take into account factors such as age, pre-existing medical or sport-related problems and what our ultimate goal is. But whatever form of exercise you choose, there are several universal principles that apply to all forms of activity.

The key points on exercise are:

1 Warm up This is something that many of us fail to do time and time again (myself included), and it leads to a significant increased risk of tendon and muscle injury. As we get older, warming up as part of any training programme becomes essential, and needs to consist of at least 5–10 minutes of mild exercise to improve blood flow and generate a cardiac response.

2 Push it This refers to what you are hoping to achieve from exercising. If it is for mental health, to take a break from work or just to improve blood flow, a gentle walk is going to be beneficial at any age; however, if your aim is to get fitter or stronger, or to decrease your CVD risk, you need to put the effort in. It does not have to be unpleasant, but for exercise to improve your physiology, it needs to make your heart rate rise, you should get out of breath and ideally your muscles should get tired.

3 Get into a routine Gym memberships always spike in January when people set a New Year's resolution to get fit, but attendance subsequently declines over the following months. For exercise to succeed in keeping us healthy, it has to be part of our weekly routine; for example, when starting to lift weights, strength might go up very quickly, but noticing an observable change in muscle size can take up to three months. When it comes to the health benefits of exercise, no matter what type of activity you choose, integrating it into your life so that it becomes part of your routine is the key to sustainability.

4 Record your progress There is a general rule of diminishing returns when it comes to exercise, and the better we get at something, the smaller the improvements we will see. Therefore, a useful way to make sure we remain on track and continue to strive to progress is to keep a record of our performance. This is true for many aerobic and strength-training activities, and with the invention of numerous training apps it can be easier to monitor our progress than ever before.

5 No excuses One of the most common excuses I hear from patients as to why they do not exercise is that they do not have time. Although I might appear unsympathetic, practically, this statement is just unacceptable. Many of us have jobs that take up more time than we would like, and some also have children or other life commitments that prevent us from taking the time for ourselves that we need. But if we do not exercise, we are doing ourselves a disservice and potentially shortening our lives and increasing our risk of multiple medical and psychological problems in the future.

6 Stay hydrated The idea that we must drink at least two litres of water every day to stay healthy is false, and there is little evidence to back this up; however, if we are significantly dehydrated, this can have a major impact on our ability to exercise and play sport. In addition, exercise itself increases our need for fluid, so my advice is to look at your urine: if it is anything darker than a light straw colour, you need to drink more.

7 Stretch Unless you are doing predominantly flexibility training, stretching is an important aspect of exercise that is often neglected. We have already established its importance in maintaining muscle health, core strength and balance, but stretching should be performed every time we train; however, do it at the end, *never* at the beginning of a session. This is because stretching cold muscles or tendons can result in a tear, whereas stretching at the end of exercise can potentially help with reducing soreness the next day.

8 What you should eat after exercise There is a myth that after training we have a one-hour window to ingest suitable amounts of protein to refuel our muscles. Although there is some evidence behind this 'protein window', it is not strictly true. Once we have exercised, our muscles are more receptive to proteins and amino acids for many hours, sometimes even up to 48 hours. This means that we have a much longer period with which we can support our muscle growth and repair than first thought. Clearly, if you exercise while fasting, the need for carbohydrates and protein replacement will be greater, and although there are small benefits to eating soon after training, we generally function well by eating every 4–5 hours, and this does not have to change with exercise.

9 Just do something The human body was never designed to be sedentary. Modern life has moved us away from our evolutionary path where once, as primitive cavemen, we would spend most of our day physically active and hunting for food, building shelter or running away from a woolly mammoth. As modern men, we are so contradictory to our evolutionary ancestors that we actually have to buy books or follow apps to remind us how to be active again. If you were to produce a lifestyle product as the ultimate all-in-one pill to improve health, it would be exercise, as countless studies have shown the enormous benefits it has on virtually all aspects of our bodies.

If all else fails

You might have lost weight, stopped smoking, started drinking alcohol-free beer, de-stressed your life and exercise three hours a day, but you might still also have high blood pressure and high cholesterol, and you might go on to develop heart disease. This is because, just as we cannot alter being men, neither can we change our genes. Although lifestyle can play an enormous role in our general health and well-being, if we are genetically prone to have high blood pressure, it might be that the only way to keep this under control is by visiting a doctor.

For many men, accepting that they might need medical intervention to prevent the onset of an illness can be tough, and it is often viewed as a failure on our part because we did not adopt a strict enough lifestyle. I still have countless patients who boast about having not seen a doctor for 20 years, or advocate taking herbal supplements in preference to a cholesterol tablet. But there is no weakness or failure in taking a medication that prevents us from becoming ill.

As men, we need to change our mindset about what we define as illness and disease in the 21st century. We need to move away from reactive medicine, whereby we wait for the problems to happen, and move towards a preventative and proactive way of thinking about our health. If your father died of a heart attack at 40, then leading a healthy lifestyle is important, but you might still require medication to keep your blood pressure within normal limits. It can be hard for many of us to accept this, but while we can make great gains in what we achieve through lifestyle measures, we have to accept that we cannot treat everything through lifestyle alone; however, by addressing these issues early in life, even if it means taking a tablet or two from a younger age, it might mean that you never have to see that cardiologist for treatment of a heart attack.

Summary

- In 2016, the WHO recorded heart disease and stroke as the world's biggest killers, accounting for a combined 15.2 million deaths worldwide.
- Men have higher rates of cardiovascular disease, high blood pressure, high cholesterol, and heart attacks and strokes than women.
- The reasons for these are multifactorial and include our DNA, our psychology and our social practices and lifestyles.
- Despite fitness and gyms becoming more mainstream, our increasingly sedentary lives and easy access to high-calorie food is causing an epidemic of obesity that is resulting in increased numbers of associated cardiovascular-related health problems.
- When it comes to weight loss, there are multiple diets available, but unless the goal is rapid weight loss, it is best to avoid diets that restrict certain foods, or radically reduce calories, as we do not know the long-term effects of these diets on our overall health. Instead, aim for a more measured style of eating, such as the Mediterranean diet.
- When it comes to exercise, everyone should be doing it. Whether it is aerobic, strength training or flexibility training, it is imperative that we find something that gets our bodies moving and increases our heart rate. We are not built to be sedentary, and although it might sound trite, exercise really is the best medicine.
- Even if you train hard and eat well, some conditions, such as high blood pressure, might not be able to be managed by lifestyle factors alone. In these cases, seeing a doctor is not a sign of failure but just that you are taking a proactive approach to your health, as prevention is always better than cure.

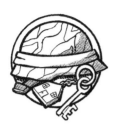

CASE STUDY

When soldiers come home

A good predictor of how easy a consultation is going to be with a patient is often inversely proportional to how many people walk into the room for a single appointment. In general, the more people, the longer and more complicated the problem is going to be. Therefore, when Raj walked in with his wife, mother and brother, I knew that this was not going to be quick. Incidentally, it is also interesting in such cases to see who in the group takes the lead; there is almost always one person who is the driver and directs the consultation in the way they want it to go. In this case, Raj's mother instantly commanded the attention of the room; although in her mid-seventies, she was sprightly, highly focused and appeared to be the sort of woman one might refer to as a 'battleaxe'.

'Thank you for agreeing to see us Dr Foster,' she said with a firm and authoritative tone.

'I am here about my son, Rajan.' She then glanced to the right as if to emphasise who she was referring to. 'As you can see by looking at him, he is struggling, and we have come to you because we don't know what else to do.'

Raj was in his early forties, was tall and lean, and had the appearance of someone who had the potential to be a great athlete but had let himself go. So far, Raj had avoided eye contact with me, looking only at the floor throughout his mother's introduction. As she went on to describe his life, the rest of the family also remained silent.

Raj had joined the army in his late teens. According to his mother, as a child he rebelled against discipline and an acceptance of rules and authority. His performance at school was average, he lacked focus, and did not know what he wanted to do as he reached the end of his education. His father (now dead) had been in the Indian Navy, and it was felt that if Raj also joined the armed forces, he might find a focus and something to be passionate about. Surprisingly, it appeared that Raj's parents were right. Although initially reluctant, Raj settled into military life well and quickly adapted to the routine and regime of being a soldier. At this point, Raj interrupted. He was well spoken and articulate, but appeared oddly disinterested in the conversation describing his own life.

'It was easy really. You didn't have to think too much,' he said. 'You're told what to do right from the off. The stupid or lazy ones fight it or leave, but the smart ones adapt, and I found it easier than being at home.'

Raj adapted so well in fact, that he quickly progressed through the ranks and ended up in the paratroopers, serving tours in the Kosovo war in 1999 and completing a tour in Afghanistan. There had obviously been other aspects to his work in the military, but Raj's mother had specifically mentioned these two conflicts in an obvious attempt to provide me with an indication of the noteworthy, front-line combat Raj had been involved in.

After more than a decade serving his country, Raj left the military when he was 34 and settled down in a small village in Warwickshire, got married, and set up a successful career as a property developer.

'A lot of people think that it's hard to adapt to civilian life when you leave the military,' Raj's mother continued, 'but actually it's just about finding a new focus and goal, and realising that life has to be different. Doesn't it, Rajan?'

She turned again to look at her son, who nodded his head slowly in agreement, while still looking at his shoes. Cracks started to appear in Raj's mental health about a year after he left the army. At first, he found it hard to sleep, started to get less focused on work and noticed he was arguing more with his wife. As his condition worsened, he went to the doctor, who had diagnosed Raj with 'stress/anxiety', and he was given a course of antidepressants. But for Raj, the tablets hadn't really helped, so he stopped them after about six weeks and, feeling dejected, never went back to the GP. Over the next year Raj began to drink heavily, initially just to help him sleep, but also to help him forget, and by the time his mother brought him to see me, his situation had deteriorated so much that he was now separated from his wife, living with his mother, his business was effectively bankrupt, and he was relying on his brother for financial support.

At this point Raj's mother stopped talking and all the family (except Raj) looked at me expectantly. It was an uncomfortable, but not unusual, scenario, where the patient or relative tells you the introduction to the story and then effectively hands it over, expecting you to finish the story by solving the problem. I knew this was where I was expected to reveal my grand plan to solve Raj's crisis, but realistically the most important thing I could do at this stage was to get everyone else except Raj and myself out of the room. Up until this point he had barely said more than a few words, and it felt like the external influences of his family – his mother in particular – were preventing Raj from expressing how he really felt.

'Mum's right in a way, everything is fine at first,' Raj said once everyone else had left the room. 'You come out and you're excited to see everyone, you have a plan, and you know what you want to do. All that other stuff is just switched off and you can put it to the back of your mind and forget about it. But that's just wishful thinking, and the novelty of being home wears off, then the same doubts and worries start to creep back into your head.'

Raj explained that he had never really been too confident, and although he was able to adapt to the regime and processes of being in the army, as he became more experienced he found some elements of conflict particularly unsettling, noticing that over time he was finding it harder and harder to resolve these doubts in his own mind. Raj was obviously reluctant to go into detail, but told me that sometimes he would have nightmares and flashbacks of particularly traumatic events, which would usually come on a few weeks before his next tour, and build with increasing regularity until he left home. But Raj never told anyone, and he never opened up to his military colleagues or even his close friends or family for fear of being seen as weak. He never told his wife, his brother or mother as they were finally happy that he had found his vocation, and he never told the army doctors, because he didn't want to get signed off sick.

'So why didn't you take the meds given to you by the GP and follow his plan?' I asked, especially concerned that there might be a similar outcome to our conversation. But Raj, now free of his family's influence, seemed much more willing to open up.

'Have you read the side effects of those things?' he asked. 'They're horrific. I slept way too much. I was never happy. Sure, I wasn't as down, but the problem was that I felt nothing. My wife said that I was like a robot. But that's not even the worst of it. It completely messed up my ability to perform in the bedroom; the pills mess up every aspect. You have no drive and then whenever we did try, I couldn't ejaculate. It got to the point where my wife thought it was her, and to be honest, I think the tablets actually made things worse for us, so I stopped taking them.'

It was easy to appreciate Raj's perspective, the pills designed to make him feel better had done nothing to improve his quality of life. He was reluctant to try other medications for fear of their side effects, and he felt scared to open up and speak to someone about his past traumas. Therefore, after much coercion, Raj tentatively agreed to talk to a psychologist I knew who specialised in post-traumatic stress disorder (PTSD), and he also agreed to trial a very mild antidepressant. This whole process was about building a relationship of trust with Raj so that he could talk about his problems and be secure enough to say if a pill worked for him or not. Over time, as his confidence in me increased, we reduced Raj's alcohol intake, got him to go to counselling with his wife, and put him in touch with the Veteran's Society for additional support. I saw Raj every two weeks for several months, until eventually he said that he felt more like his old self; he moved back in with his wife, stopped relying on his brother for money, and was able to attend the appointments unaccompanied, without the assistance of his mother. The outcome appeared good.

Every case study I have written about in this book has been a real patient I have seen at some stage in my career. As such, the stories tend not to fit a conventional narrative, and Raj is no different. Our first consultation, the one described above, happened five years ago, and despite his initial improvement, Raj relapsed a few months later. He stopped engaging with me, started drinking heavily again, and his wife moved out. Despite referring him to psychologists, counsellors and psychiatrists, and trying multiple medications, Raj's story does not conclude with either a terrible tragedy or a rise to success and happiness. Just like many PTSD sufferers, Raj was never 'fixed' – he just keeps going.

I now see Raj only when his depression or anxiety get on top of him, or when he falls off the wagon. Sometimes he comes alone, sometimes with his ex-wife, or when things are really bad, he sees me with his mother. The rest of the time, Raj struggles on, trying to keep his business afloat, to remain close to his family and maintain some illusion of normality. We know mental illness affects people in different ways, but for men who have been raised and trained to be tough and resilient it can be particularly hard for them to accept the need for help. The fear of failure, or being seen as weak in the eyes of their peers can make it almost impossible for soldiers (or any highly driven person) to ask for help. In the modern world men are still encouraged to be strong and resilient. When they are young, boys are told not to cry, and if they are hurt, 'don't be girl'. On the other hand, we are constantly telling men that they need to talk about their feelings and should be comfortable opening up about their fears and anxieties with friends and family. Perhaps more than any other mental illness, PTSD illustrates the opposing positions men are faced with when trying to find a way to fit in today's society.

CHAPTER 3

Mental Health

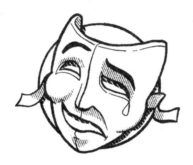

W e all know someone who has struggled with their mental health, and in fact the number of people diagnosed with a mental illness globally is increasing year on year. According to the WHO, there are approximately 264 million people worldwide suffering with depression. In the UK approximately 4 million men (one in eight) suffer from some form of mental illness,[1] with the majority of suicides being male. Recently, there have been substantial efforts made to provide better awareness of mental health and reduce some of the stigma surrounding this area of medicine. We have seen many high-profile celebrities and actors talking openly about their struggles with mental health. In addition, new charities have been created, and there is now a wealth of online support for people wishing to know more about the symptoms, causes and treatment of mental illness.

Despite efforts made to raise awareness of mental health, for many men talking about their feelings or worries still remains a taboo subject. This means that they are not seeking help, and consequently many men do not get the support and treatment they need. Although the prevalence of the more common mental illnesses such as depression and anxiety is actually higher in women, the Samaritans suicide statistics report from 2018 found that in the UK there were 6,507 suicides, of which approximately 75 per cent were men aged between 45 and 49.[2] This was a rise of 10 per cent compared with the previous year. Most concerning, however, is that high numbers of male suicide are a repeated statistic that occurs year on year.

To make matters worse, the global coronavirus pandemic of 2020 has resulted in a huge increase in the number of patients wanting to access mental-health treatment and support. The forced reduction in social interaction, economic downturn, delay in medical services and the relentless fear-provoking news coverage has not only caused those with existing mental-health problems to relapse, but provoked anxiety in people who have never suffered with mental illness before.

Irrespective of the hopefully temporary effect of Covid-19, high-profile celebrity and media campaigns to encourage men to talk openly, and more information and support for mental health being available than ever before, men are still responsible for three-quarters of suicides, and this figure has persisted for more than ten years. This chapter aims to look at why mental-health outcomes remain poor for men, why male-orientated psychology and psychiatry remain such a difficult area of health to improve, and what you can do if you think you might be suffering with mental illness.

The history of mental illness

We now live in a world where the majority of us do not worry about basic survival. We have food, water, warmth, security and a complex and supportive social structure. This means that we are now better off than all our descendants ever were and in ways that they could not imagine. We do not worry about where we will get our next meal or being attacked by wild animals; we have warm, safe houses, sanitation, vaccinations and advances in medicine, meaning that we live longer and healthier lives. Now, more than at any point in human history, we are better off, and as a consequence we should be happier and more content. Yet this is not reflected in the numbers of people suffering with depression and other forms of mental illness. If depression and anxiety are primarily triggered by adverse life events, such as disease, disability, poverty and other life-impacting problems, it seems bizarre that the numbers of people being diagnosed with mental illness keep increasing. Obviously, we need to take into account a better awareness of mental health by the general population and diagnosis by doctors, but even taking these factors into account, the massive impact that mental illness has on societies globally suggests that it is more complex than just a series of external triggers that affect how we feel.

Mental illness is not a new problem, and as far back as 400BC, Hippocrates used the term 'melancholia' to describe people who suffered from problems with their mental health. Melancholia was an umbrella term used to describe virtually all forms of psychiatric disorders, from severe sadness and anxiety to hallucinations, delusions and psychosis. And, like all aspects of medicine and disease at this time, Hippocrates believed that a deficiency in, or more commonly an excess of, one of the four essential bodily fluids (humours) – blood, yellow bile, black bile and phlegm – was responsible for all physical and mental disease. Melancholia, in particular, was usually associated with abnormalities in black bile, and treatment for this condition could vary from medicines to affect the bowel or even the release of excess blood (known as bloodletting). Astonishingly, humourism remained an important element in medicine and health up until the 19th century.

As barbaric as bloodletting might appear for the treatment of mental (or any) illness, the ancient Greek physicians had made a breakthrough in psychiatric medicine by suggesting that diseases originated either from problems within the body or as a result of external triggers. This enlightened way of thinking was in stark contrast to the dominant theory of the time, which suggested that supernatural spirits or demonic possession caused physical or mental illness. Many orthodox religions perpetuated this idea, and even up until the 15th century it was generally accepted that mental illness occurred as a result of witchcraft or the influence of the devil.

In the 16th century, specific institutions known as asylums were created to care for people whose mental illness was thought to be so severe that they posed a risk to themselves or others. For many years, these institutions remained uncommon, but the 18th century saw a rapid rise in the building and development of 'mental asylums'. Prior to this, mental illness was viewed primarily as a domestic problem, with families and churches being responsible for the majority of care. Occasionally, if local support was not available, patients could be committed to private 'madhouses', or taken on by other members of the community. Initially, it was only those patients who were at distinct risk of being violent or were particularly disturbed who were confined to the asylums.

Most inmates of asylums were institutionalised against their will and often lived in filth, chained to walls and exhibited to the public for a fee. The understanding of mental-health problems during the establishment of the asylums was particularly poor, and it was widely thought that those with severe mental illness were similar to animals in that they lacked capacity and the ability to reason. As a result, patients in asylums were not given the same rights as the 'sane'. A common theory was that by instilling fear into patients, it would help to restore a disordered mind back to reason. Unsurprisingly, success rates for this type of therapy were low, but as asylums continued to multiply in Europe and North America in the 1800s, psychiatry became a recognised medical speciality. Since the establishment of the asylums in the 16th century, understanding the causes and triggers of mental illness had improved very little. But by building and populating asylums it provided doctors with an interest in mental health, with a relatively constant influx of new patients to examine. As psychology and psychiatry became established disciplines, a better understanding of mental illness followed.

Although the psychology of mental health had improved, it wasn't really until the development of antidepressants in the 1980s that psychiatric medicines became available to mass groups of patients. Prior to this, although antipsychotics had found limited success in the treatment of mental illness, other forms of treatment largely relied on tranquillisers, electroconvulsive (electroshock) therapy or even lobotomy. It was the release of antidepressants as a widely available, cheap and effective drug that allowed doctors to treat more patients than ever before, and consequently the numbers of people diagnosed with mental illness rapidly started to increase.

Are we supposed to be happy?

Most people with mental-health problems I see in clinic tend to suffer with either depression or anxiety, or a mixture of both. Patients with these milder forms of mental illness tend not to require hospital admission, they will never see a psychiatrist and commonly have not suffered from severe traumatic life events that could be a trigger for their condition. But despite this, the prevalence of the less severe forms of mental illness is rising. Films, TV and social media, in particular, have presented an image of what we think our lives should be like. Even in children's fairy tales, the term 'they lived happily ever after' is a recurrent theme that we are led to believe should apply to our own lives from childhood. But we all know that happiness is temporary, and from an evolutionary perspective are we even supposed to be happy?

Perhaps the first mistake in deciding if we are engineered to be happy is to presume that evolution has any role in it. When it comes to the basic concept of our reason for existence, we are no different from other animals. From an evolutionary perspective, all we need to do is survive in our environment for long enough so that we can reproduce and briefly ensure that the next generation does the same. Whether we are happy or content during this process is basically irrelevant. A constant state of contentment or happiness would in fact be counterproductive, as it would reduce our anxiety about potential threats and decrease our drive to find a new mate. Humans' brains have developed a large frontal lobe that allows us to use language. It facilitates improved problem solving and better motor function as well as developed social and sexual behaviour, plus many other higher intellectual functions; however, the increased development of our brains has not improved our ability to stay happy. Therefore, although depression and anxiety are not simply the absence of happiness, it is important to understand that as a species it is normal for us to suffer with low mood, to feel stress and ruminate over problems, and not to be consistently joyful.

To say that happiness is irrelevant to our existence,

however, is obviously an oversimplification. Certainly, being happy is beneficial and is something we are always striving to achieve. Happiness helps us to find and keep mates, it improves social cohesion and it has numerous physiological and psychological benefits, such as reducing stress and the risk of heart disease, while boosting our immune system, and it might even increase our life expectancy. Therefore, happiness should be best viewed as something transient, and we must appreciate that being sad, negative or stressed does not mean that we have failed or have a mental illness, but it is just a normal part of being human.

Risk factors for mental illness, depression and anxiety

Unlike physical illness, where common diseases have certain triggers, which result in a certain disease, the causes and risk factors for the development of mental illnesses are far less straightforward. To make a diagnosis in mental health, doctors rely on a series of behavioural symptoms and signs, which can be the result of events that might have occurred at any point in a person's life. To make matters worse, traumatic life events affect people differently, and we don't always know why one person is less able than another to cope with a stressful event. We do know that there are established risk factors that, cumulatively, make the likelihood of developing mental illness greater, and these risk factors can be divided into four main areas.

Social and environmental factors

Social and environmental pressures can occur in any aspect of our lives and are common contributors to a decline in mental health; for example, I see many patients attending the clinic with stress brought on by work pressures. Typically, men describe feeling trapped in their job, often with unsupportive management and a loss of autonomy. Over time, their stress levels increase until they can no longer cope and they suffer a true anxiety disorder. Financial hardship is another factor in the development of stress, because the fear of increasing debt, and its implications on housing, food and family, can make patients acutely unwell. Relationship stresses, such as divorce, can also trigger a decline in mental health, and in many cases, relationship breakups are made worse for men by the social isolation that occurs when they are removed from the family home and might be denied access to their children.

Post-traumatic stress disorder (PTSD) is perhaps the best illustration of how environmental factors can result in mental illness. Although we now have a good understanding of what causes PTSD, and who is at risk of developing it, it wasn't until 1980 that it was formally recognised as a psychiatric condition. PTSD is a mental illness brought on primarily by an experience that is overwhelming, frightening and beyond our control. This can develop after a car accident, being the victim of an assault or through having a high-risk job that is likely to involve exposure to extreme psychological trauma. PTSD is, therefore, commonly seen in people who work for the emergency services and in the military.

Finally, one of the biggest environmental risk factors for the development of mental illness is the use, and more commonly abuse, of alcohol and drugs. For some people, drinking alcohol or taking drugs is a method by which they try to cope with the emerging symptoms of mental illness. This is known as 'self-medicating', but in conjunction with the physical damage drugs and alcohol cause, prolonged self-medicating actually makes mental-health outcomes worse. For most people, the initial benefit of 'being able to forget', or 'blocking out voices', is short-lived, as users tend to develop tolerance to the drug and therefore require ever-increasing amounts to gain the same benefits. Alcohol is itself a depressant, and, just like many other drugs, chronic use can result in a deterioration of mood as well as reducing the effects of antidepressant medications.

For some people, taking drugs and alcohol, while hoping to improve their mental health, can actually make their conditions worse. The possible long-term effects of drug and alcohol use include:

- Tolerance (as discussed above)
- Dependence (craving the drug without getting any benefit or high)
- Withdrawal symptoms, if you stop using the drug
- Decreased motivation, energy and drive
- Negative impact on relationships with family and friends
- Worsening depression
- Difficulty maintaining a job

- Getting into debt
- Developing drug-induced psychosis

Even more worryingly, there is now good evidence that some drugs, such as cannabis, can actually trigger the onset of mental illnesses such as psychosis and schizophrenia.[3] The younger patients are when they begin to use cannabis, the greater they are at risk of developing the illness due to the fact that their brains are still developing.

Finally, it is worth noting that many medications that are used to treat mental illness are less effective when combined with drugs or alcohol. Therefore, not only can taking drugs or alcohol make mental-health symptoms worse but they can also reduce the effectiveness of treatment. This poses a particularly difficult challenge for doctors and other health professionals where patients are heavily reliant on recreational drugs when they start a treatment plan.

Psychological factors

Psychological risk factors for the development of mental illness include bereavement, difficulties in relating to other people, handling stress badly, and any mental trauma, in particular, abuse. Adult and child abuse, whether emotional, physical, sexual or neglect, are powerful triggers for the onset of mental illness, and victims tend to be more prone to anxiety, depression, PTSD, drug abuse, addiction and personality disorders. In severe cases, abuse can even lead to patients developing dissociative identity disorder (formally known as multiple personality disorder), where patients take on at least two distinct personalities.

For many victims of child abuse, the events are so traumatic that they will stunt normal psychological development. Fear of cruelty or mistreatment prevents abused children from being able to form the normal attachments with parents or other family members that are required for us to interact socially and form healthy relationships as adults. In severe cases, early childhood trauma can be so devastating that it can even result in trouble remembering daily tasks, learning new things or making simple decisions as an adult. In an attempt to manage their abuse some people will compartmentalise the events and effectively block out the trauma from their day-to-day lives. As a consequence, however, a specific trigger many years on might cause them to relive aspects of their abuse and bring on the onset of a new mental illness. In addition to the effect that deliberate psychological trauma might have on the developing mind, major early losses, such as the death of a parent or loved one, might also result in long-term attachment problems, confidence and trust issues, and eventually present as depression.

Obviously, it is not surprising that being the victim of abuse, or losing a parent, is likely to lead to mental-health problems as an adult; however, it is important to emphasise that traumatic events do not have to be that severe to result in changes in psychological growth and a healthy adult mind. Indeed, we might all have mildly traumatic experiences that we went through as children that were not necessarily abusive, but which might have altered our psychological resilience as adults.

Genetics

In the last decade, there has been considerable research looking into the links between mental health and genetics, and it is now accepted that certain genes or genetic variations are associated with an increased risk of developing mental illness. Typical psychiatric conditions that tend to have a genetic component include autism, attention deficit hyperactivity disorder (ADHD), bipolar disorder, major depression and schizophrenia.[4]

The inherited risk of developing mental illness has particular impact when looking at asymptomatic people who might have family members already suffering with a mental-health condition, or if someone themselves has a mental illness and is worried about passing it on to their children.

Although there are many mental illnesses with a genetic component, it is important to stress that the presence of a variant gene is never enough in itself to predict if someone will go on to develop a mental illness. To complicate things further, the isolated presence of a specific gene cannot even tell us what the percentage risk of getting a mental illness might be. This is because of the multifactorial nature of mental health, and because there is no such thing as one straightforward gene 'for' complex traits like mental health disorders. Inheritance is always a game of probability and not destiny. This is also why home genetic testing is so dangerous. All genetic testing can do is tell you the presence, or absence, of a specific gene. It offers us nothing in terms of risk. Testing can falsely reassure us, but equally it can incorrectly worry us.

When looking at genes in psychiatric conditions, it is crucial to stress that although there is a genetic link in mental illness, this is only one contributing factor from a large list of social, psychological and biological causes.

Biological risk factors

Physical disease is intrinsically linked to mental illness, but when we look at how these two conditions affect each other, it is important to separate those physical conditions that directly cause a change in mental state and those that are so disabling that they cause a decline in our mental health. The reason for this differentiation is that chronic physical disability is really a psychological risk factor for mental illness, rather than something that directly affects our brains' ability to function normally. The impact that chronic physical illness can have on mental health is now so well established that the British National Institute for Health and Care Excellence (NICE) has advised that doctors and nurses should be aware of the risk of depression in any patient with a disabling physical problem and especially those with a history of depression.[5] NICE advises that clinicians should be asking patients two simple questions:

1. During the last month, have you often been bothered by feeling down, depressed or hopeless?
2. During the last month, have you often been bothered by having little interest or pleasure in doing things?

Clearly, these questions in themselves are not sufficient to diagnose a mental illness, but they are a quick and effective screening tool that can raise the possibility that a patient might be suffering from depression. It is quite understandable that patients who are suffering long-term disability through physical disease are more likely to feel low and suffer with depression; however, it is only relatively recently that the questions mentioned above have been asked due, in part, to our increasing knowledge and understanding of the interactions between body and mind.

In terms of looking at how physical disease can directly result in mental illness, a WHO study in 2007 looked at 245,400 patients in 60 countries and found that those with two or more chronic physical health problems experienced a prevalence of depression of 23 per cent.[6] Although some conditions, such as an underactive thyroid gland, are known to cause changes in mood, the range of diseases and concerns that can cause an altered mental state is large. Some common examples of medical conditions that can mimic mental illness, or cause changes in mental state, include:

- Neurological causes
- Multiple sclerosis, Parkinson's disease, Alzheimer's disease and Huntington's disease
- Vascular causes
- Stroke
- Nutritional deficiencies
- Vitamin B12 or vitamin D deficiency
- Hormonal disorders
- Thyroid, parathyroid or adrenal gland disease

- Sex hormone deficiencies
- Testosterone deficiency in men, and menopause in women
- Certain immune-system diseases such as lupus
- Certain infections, such as glandular fever, hepatitis and HIV
- Certain cancers
- Prescribed medications
- Certain medications, such as antimalarial tablets, anti-inflammatory steroids such as prednisolone or anabolic steroid abuse

It is worth noting that it is rare for the conditions listed above to cause changes in mental health without any associated physical symptoms, but it is useful to be aware of just how many medical problems can alter our mental health. It is also a useful reminder that we should never focus solely on the physical symptoms of disease.

When does extreme emotion become mental illness?

As the number of people with mental-health problems continues to rise, it is important to distinguish between what is true mental illness and what is just a state of being sad. This confusion can lead to more serious illnesses being missed, or, equally, an overreaction and medicalisation of a normal emotional state. Although the latter might lead to unnecessary medical or psychological treatment, the former could have serious consequences in terms of the overall health and safety of a patient.

The key elements of sadness and stress are that they are normal human emotions. Everyone experiences them, but they are usually short-lived and have a clear trigger; for example, the triggers for sadness tend to be events that are upsetting, disappointing or hurtful, whereas the triggers for stress tend to be the presence of high-pressure, tense or important experiences that have significant implications or potential outcomes. It is our ability to approach these problems rationally, using support networks to reflect on bad experiences, that allows us to move on and return to a normal emotional state.

Depression and anxiety are different. In these conditions, there is an abnormal emotional state that affects our ability to function on a day-to-day basis. Depression and anxiety can affect every aspect of our lives, including our ability to concentrate, our memory, emotions, perception of others, and our physical health in terms of sleep, appetite, energy and general well-being. Furthermore, these feelings are enduring and long-lasting, and our ability to reflect and rationalise is lost. In depression, in particular, there might be no specific trigger or terrible life event, which can make it even harder for patients to feel that they can talk about their feelings. I have seen countless patients with depression who feel guilty for suffering with their condition because they have had good lives and 'should' be happy.

When trying to understand if the normal emotions of sadness and stress have become a true mental illness, it is useful to recognise that depression and anxiety affect every aspect of a patient's life. This includes their ability to love or feel loved, to feel happiness or enjoyment in any activity,

to be able to cope with simple tasks such as going to buy
groceries, in interactions with strangers or even the ability
to wash and dress. In major depression, patients can suffer
such a complete lack of motivation and energy that even
getting out of bed becomes impossible.

Because of the complexity of mental illness, and the fact
that there is no single identifying test, diagnoses of depression and anxieties are defined by thresholds. In practice this
means having five of the following symptoms for at least
two weeks:

1. A depressed or irritable mood most of the time.
2. A loss or decrease of pleasure or interest in most
    activities, including ones that had been interesting
    or pleasurable previously.
3. Significant increases or decreases in weight
    or appetite.
4. Sleeping too much or sleeping too little compared
    with usual.
5. Feeling restless or anxious, or that you have slowed
    down in your movements.
6. Feeling tired, having no energy or motivation
    most days.
7. Feeling worthless, or having feelings of exces-
    sive guilt.
8. Experiencing decreases in mental acuity, such as
    problems with memory, focus or concentration, or
    the ability to make decisions.
9. Thoughts of suicide or making plans to die.

It is worth stressing that while these points are useful tools as an aid in making a diagnosis of depression, they are still only one part of an overall assessment and should always be considered as part of a wider picture of a patient's health.

Why is suicide greater in men?

As we have seen, suicide remains the biggest cause of death of men under the age of 45 in the UK. The suicide rate remains at about 15.5 deaths per 100,000 for men and 4.9 deaths per 100,000 for women,[7] which means that approximately 75 per cent of suicides are male. But this statistic is not restricted to the UK. Globally, there are no countries where women are more likely to commit suicide than men.

Despite the fact that the vast majority of suicides globally are male, more women actually suffer with depression and are nearly twice as likely to suffer from anxiety. In fact, when looking at depression and anxiety, one in five women suffer symptoms, compared with only one in eight men. Not only do more women suffer with mental-health problems but also they are more likely to attempt suicide, more likely to discuss having suicidal thoughts and exhibit suicidal behaviour. Therefore, if more women suffer with mental illness, express the desire to kill themselves and try to commit suicide more often, why is the death rate greater in men?

One reason for the difference in male to female suicide rates is that men tend to commit suicide through more violent and calculated methods. Women will often, not necessarily consciously, choose a method of suicide that is

potentially treatable or reversible, such as taking an over-
dose. Men, on the other hand, tend to choose more violent
methods of suicide, such as jumping from a height, using
firearms or hanging. These methods are far more commit-
tal, and once the suicidal attempt is initiated, it is often
impossible for other people to help or intervene.

It is not entirely clear why men choose more violent
methods of suicide, but several theories exist, including
the idea that men are simply more intent on dying. Women
have been shown to reach out for help more when they
are depressed or suicidal, and it has been suggested that a
higher proportion of suicide attempts in women are actually
cries for help. This is probably a reflection of the fact that,
in general, men are considered to have a more 'black and
white' approach to their thinking, whereas women tend to
view problems as 'shades of grey'. As such, whether at a
conscious or unconscious level, women are able to think
more insightfully about their mental health and ask for help.

Another theory behind the aggressive nature of male
suicide is that men tend to act more instinctively to situations rather than thinking first and acting later. This can
mean that male suicidal behaviour is more spontaneous and
does not allow for reflection, consideration of loved ones,
or other options that could possibly stop the suicide from
going ahead. It is common for men to act more impulsively
than women in many aspects of life, and although only a
generalisation, women tend to take their time and think
about a problem more before they take action. When this
male impulsivity is applied to suicide attempts, the outcomes understandably will be more severe.

One of the most curious theories around the method used in suicide is that women tend to choose a way that preserves their appearance, and avoids facial disfigurement.[8] The theory is interesting because it suggests that even when it comes to suicide, men and women act out culturally prescribed gender roles. Although the evidence for this theory is less well established, a study of 621 suicides in Ohio (North America) found that when both sexes used firearms to commit suicide women were less likely to shoot themselves in the head.[9]

Apart from the method used, there are several societal and psychological factors that increase the risk of male suicide. Traditional gender stereotypes discourage men from expressing their emotions; for example, from an early age we tell children that 'big boys don't cry' and that they should be tough, but we encourage girls to be open about their feelings. Despite promoting a more open society towards talking about male mental health, we are still conditioning boys from a young age that they should be strong and silent about their emotions and that they should not demonstrate weakness by crying. This burying of emotions, and pressure not to demonstrate weakness or failure, is inevitably going to produce adult males who feel unable to speak to loved ones about their worries or feelings. This is reflected in the fact that when women suffer with mental-health problems, they are more likely to ask for help from friends, colleagues and family than men. Sadly, for the majority of men, the concept of the British 'stiff upper lip' still applies and has resulted in a culture that prevents many men from feeling able to speak to their doctor, or anyone else, about their mental health.

As a consequence of men asking for help less frequently, it is highly likely that the true numbers of people suffering with depression are actually far greater. It usually takes a man several visits to their GP for them to be able to express how bad they really feel, and this is consistent with the theory discussed above, suggesting that men are programmed from a young age to suppress their emotions, and that admitting that they are struggling is a sign of weakness. Because men are less likely to seek help in the early stages of mental illness, it often leads to higher drug and alcohol use, a worsening of mental illness and a subsequent increased risk of suicide.

What can I do if I think I might be suffering with a mental illness?

In the UK, men are still only about half as likely as women to access psychological therapies, and we know that they are less likely to speak to family or friends about their mental health. In younger men in particular, there is also a harmful trend to turn to dangerous coping methods such as drug or alcohol abuse. Therefore, the first, and most important, thing to do if you feel you might be starting to struggle with your mental health is to speak to someone. This does not have to be anyone medically trained, and actually, in the early stages of most mental illnesses, opening up to family or friends can make a big difference to how you feel. This simple step of talking more openly can help break the male stigma and social pressure to internalise our problems, and it can be a crucial way of helping to reduce a deterioration in mental health.

Other ways to help improve your mental health is through online resources. In general, I try to discourage the use of Internet forums and social media, as these tend to show the more negative or destructive experiences seen in mental health, but there are numerous charities and official websites that can provide positive guidance and online psychology and support for those wishing to get help there. Many of the official sites also provide useful telephone numbers and advise ways to access local or national mental-health support services. In addition to online support and talking more openly, making personal lifestyle changes have been shown to not only improve how you feel about yourself but also to help improve outcomes in mental illnesses.

Lifestyle changes

The importance that lifestyle measures can have on our mental health is often under-recognised as they are seen as minor, trivial or insignificant; however, in virtually all mental illnesses, especially depression, lifestyle changes are a powerful tool in improving symptoms and outcome. The examples below are not exhaustive, but they help to illustrate some of the ways that improving your lifestyle can benefit your mental health.

Exercise is particularly beneficial when it comes to mental well-being. In addition to releasing the body's own feel-good chemicals, serotonin and endorphins, exercise is a metabolic stimulant that enhances blood flow and general health, and it improves brain function and mood. In 2017, a systematic review highlighted that virtually all randomised controlled trials published between 1999 and 2016 found that regular exercise helps in the treatment of depression.[10] Additionally, the exercise we do to improve our mental health does not have to be extreme. In accordance with the benefits of exercise for physical health, the advice for mental health is the same: 30–60 minutes of moderate activity on most days. (See pages 86–94 for more about exercise.)

Social isolation has been identified as a key risk factor for the development of mental illness. In many men, as their mental health declines, they enter into a negative spiral that actually promotes a desire to self-isolate further. By doing so, it initially improves anxiety and the social pressure by reducing the need to have to 'perform' and be happy around others. But as the social isolation continues, it becomes a very destructive component in deteriorating mental health. Although this compulsion to avoid social interaction can be difficult to challenge, keeping regular contact with your friends or family, or joining a club, sport or class, can help you to break the negative cycle of social isolation early and reduce the progression of mental illness.

Eating well will obviously help promote physical health, but there is also increasing evidence that a good diet can benefit our mental well-being, too. Eating a Mediterranean diet (a diet high in vegetables, fruits, legumes, nuts, beans, grains, fish and unsaturated fats such as olive oil, as described on page 84), as well as supplementing with fish oil, has been shown to decrease depression symptoms for many months after the dietary change. Furthermore, studies have also found that diets with high levels of saturated fat, refined carbohydrates (quick-release sugars) and processed foods are linked to poorer mental health in children and adolescents.[11] There are also links between mental illness and obesity, but in terms of obesity and depression it is not clear whether obesity is the cause of the depression in some patients or the depression itself leads to an increased risk of becoming obese. When trying to link diet to mental illness, it is important not to confuse correlation with causation. This is the idea that one problem might directly lead to another (causation), or it could simply be that two problems are seen together but are not related (correlation). Many people who have poor diets, low in fruit and vegetables, and a poor understanding of what is good nutrition, also have other health inequalities that are likely to contribute to a greater risk of mental illness. These are known as confounding factors, extra variables that can influence a test result, and which make a direct link between diet and mental health difficult to prove. These confounding factors include poorer physical health, living in poverty or deprived communities, drug and alcohol use, and less education with respect to healthy eating.

Sleep is vital for emotional stability, so much so that sleep deprivation can drastically affect your mental health. This is commonly seen in people who do shift work, or have newborn children. As many of us who have children will recall, this partial insomnia often leads to irritability, being short-tempered, and having poor memory and concentration.

In mental illness, poor sleep can be a cause and a consequence of worsening psychological symptoms. If you suffer
with chronic insomnia, not only does your mental health
deteriorate but also your physical health, with insomniacs
also being at an increased risk of high blood pressure and
heart disease. (See pages 33–35 for more about sleep.)

Visit your doctor

If changes to lifestyle fail to improve your symptoms, or you
are worried that you have a more serious mental illness, the
next step should be to visit your doctor. For many patients
with mental-health issues, visiting their GP can act as a
form of reflective counselling, even without prescribing any
medication or providing any formal psychological therapy.
By being objective and disconnected from a patient's social
network, it can allow men to discuss issues that they might
feel uncomfortable talking about to their friends or family.
If it looks as if further treatment options are needed, these
tend to be either talking therapies, medication or a combination of both.

What are talking therapies?

Talking therapies is a collective term used to describe a variety of psychological treatments that range from counselling
to psychotherapy. In essence, all talking therapies involve
speaking to a trained professional about how you feel, your
thoughts and your behaviour. Although the approach might
be different depending on the type of therapy used, there

are certain commonalities found in every type of talking therapy. The principles of talking therapies are:

- To provide someone with a safe environment in which they can speak openly and comfortably about their mental health without fear of embarrassment or being judged.
- To help someone gain a better understanding of themselves and why they have certain emotions that they might feel they cannot control.
- To resolve difficult or complicated emotional issues, or to provide a framework so that they can control their mental-health problems in day-to-day life, rather than their mental illness controlling them.
- To help someone gain insight into their own personality, to recognise negative patterns of behaviour and to progressively learn to manage or change them.

When looking at talking therapies, one difficulty patients commonly describe is working out which talking therapy is best suited to them, especially as there are clearly common elements that apply to them all.

Counselling usually refers to a brief treatment that centres on behavioural patterns. When patients attend their appointment, they are encouraged to talk about how they feel, their emotions, or any particular traumatic events. A counsellor can help to make sense of how we feel, as well as providing tools and plans to help patients resolve their own problems. As a patient will be discussing highly personal and emotional issues, it is essential that any therapist used is trained appropriately and registered with the Accredited Professional Standards Agency.

Psychotherapy The principles around how talking therapy works and the importance of professional accreditation applies to psychotherapy in the same way that it applies to counselling; however, psychotherapy takes longer and is more immersive than counselling, and it focuses on individuals gaining a better insight into their own emotional problems and difficulties. It tries to equip patients with the means to then change these negative behaviours so that they can better manage and control their own mental health in the future. In practice, this means understanding why someone feels or displays certain emotions, and then teaching them ways to manage or change these feelings in a positive way. There is a wide variety of psychotherapies available, but some common forms include:

- PSYCHOANALYTIC THERAPY focuses on unconscious, suppressed thoughts often stemming from childhood. Therapists encourage patients to say whatever is going on in their mind to help them become more aware of hidden patterns or behaviours that might be contributing to their mental-health problems.
- PSYCHODYNAMIC THERAPY is similar in approach to psychoanalytic therapy and focuses on how unconscious thoughts or emotions might affect the way in which we act.

- COGNITIVE BEHAVIOURAL THERAPY (CBT) looks at how specific beliefs and thoughts are linked to our behaviour and feelings. It then teaches the patient specific skills to retrain that behaviour gradually and to help to manage or control stressful situations better.
- DIALECTICAL BEHAVIOUR THERAPY (DBT) is a type of CBT, and focuses more on those who suffer with very intense emotions. It teaches patients to understand how two things that seem opposite could both be true; for example, changing your behaviour but simultaneously accepting yourself for who you are.
- COGNITIVE ANALYTICAL THERAPY (CAT) combines both psychodynamic psychotherapy and CBT to help determine why someone's specific behaviour results in problems, and how to resolve or improve them.
- MINDFULNESS is a popular form of therapy, similar to meditation. It helps someone become more aware of their thoughts and emotions, and how to accept them.
- INTERPERSONAL PSYCHOTHERAPY (IPT) is used particularly for people suffering with PTSD, as it looks at the way that specific events involving relationships, bereavements or traumas can result in changes in behaviour. It then teaches ways to cope with the associated feelings involved and provides coping strategies.
- HUMANISTIC THERAPIES encourage a patient to think about themselves more positively and to focus

on a more holistic approach looking at body, mind and even spirit.

- FAMILY AND COUPLE (SYSTEMIC) THERAPY involves therapy within a group dynamic, usually with other members of the same household, to resolve problems together.

The above list is not exhaustive, and many therapists may use additional techniques or combinations of therapies to improve outcomes for patients. When it comes to talking therapies, the key elements required for success are to make sure that the most effective form of therapy is used for that individual, making sure the patient and therapist get on well together and, most importantly, that the patient feels able to talk openly about his emotional state, feelings and past psychological history. It is this third aspect that can be particularly challenging for men who might not feel able to open up to a stranger about their insecurities or woes.

Medical therapies

In addition to talking therapies, some men might initially prefer to try using medication. There is still some stigma around antidepressants, and one common reason men state that they do not seek help for their mental health earlier is the fear of being put on antidepressants straight away. In practice, antidepressants are only one type of medication we use to treat mental illness, and others include non-addictive anti-anxiety medicines such as beta-blockers, short-term use of sleeping tablets and stronger medications issued by psychiatrists (such as antipsychotics and lithium). Even within antidepressants, there is a wide range of different types, and although there are preferred antidepressants for specific conditions, quite often it is more about finding the right medication that suits the individual.

By far the most famous antidepressant is Prozac, which was first released in 1988. Prior to its introduction, anti-depressants (such as amitriptyline and imipramine) were available but had significant side effects, as well as adverse cardiac risks. In 1975, when Prozac (drug name fluoxetine) was originally invented, it was not expected to be particu-larly successful, but it was eventually granted approval for the treatment of major depression in 1987. By 1990, Prozac had become the most widely used antidepressant of all time.

The success of Prozac comes from the fact that it is highly effective at improving mood, with very few side effects. It is a member of a family of drugs known as selective serotonin reuptake inhibitors (SSRIs). Serotonin is a chemical released between nerve cells that has a wide variety of functions in the human body including effects to the gut, bone density, clotting and how happy we feel. SSRIs work by blocking (inhibiting) reuptake of serotonin, meaning that more of it remains available to pass messages between nearby nerve cells, and it potentially makes us feel happier.

Myth buster: true or false?

Myth: antidepressants will make you happy

False. Antidepressants can reduce the symptoms of depression and anxiety, but they work by helping you to handle your emotional responses better. They can't make someone euphoric, but you might be able to cope with the stresses and challenges of life better.

Since the development of Prozac, a range of other SSRIs have been released that specifically focus on treating anxiety, depression or a combination of both. Although some people might experience the adverse side effects of SSRIs, such as nausea, feeling more anxious, dry mouth or erectile dysfunction, for the vast majority of patients who take SSRIs they have been a game changer in the way that we manage and treat mental illness.

Combining therapies

Although mental illness can often be treated with either talking therapies or medication, most patients tend to do best by using a combination of the two. This is commonly illustrated in PTSD, where many men feel uncomfortable about opening up to a therapist due to repressed experiences or memories. By taking an antidepressant, it can help them to cope with the challenges of therapy more easily and therefore assist them in addressing traumatic topics and achieve a better outcome for their mental health.

In the last ten years, there have been great advances made in attitudes towards male mental health. In addition, our understanding and treatment of mental illness as a whole has also improved significantly; however, outcomes for men remain poor, and male suicide rates continue to lag behind the improvements we see in other areas of mental health. Although medical services are treating more patients than ever before, it is only by addressing how men perceive their own mental health, and how this is reflected in society, that we are really going to improve the stigma still associated with male mental illness. We need to provide a platform that allows men to retain their sense of masculinity, without falling back into the stereotyped role of the early 20th century where men kept a stiff upper lip and buried their emotions deep inside. We can all play our part in opening up more to friends, family and work colleagues, and by teaching our children that it is okay for boys to show emotion, and for men to cry.

Summary

- Mental illness is common: one in eight men suffer with some form of mental health problem.
- Unlike physical illnesses, causes are often multifactorial and are often due to a combination of physical, psychological or social problems.
- Globally women suffer with greater levels of depression, but in every country recorded, men have a higher rate of suicide.

→

- Despite significant efforts by high-profile celebrities to break the stigma of male mental illness, we remain in a society where being a man means not talking about our feelings.
- Treatment for many forms of mental illness is successful but requires a holistic approach:

  1 Talk to a friend or family member about how you are feeling.
  2 Make sure your body is healthy by eating a good diet and exercising regularly.
  3 Develop a good sleep pattern.
  4 Engage in social activities, even if they initially make you feel uncomfortable.
  5 Avoid recreational drugs, including alcohol.

- If things fail to improve, speak to your doctor. Additional treatments include talking therapies, medications or referral to a psychiatrist.

Attitudes towards men's health are slowly changing. Help is available through various sources, and we no longer need to bury our fears and concerns. Male mental health is not something we should be ashamed to discuss.

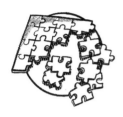

CASE STUDY

Dementia and letting go

It is commonly assumed that couples who are together in their twilight years must be happy and content because they have stayed together for so long; however, although time might provide acceptance, it is no guarantee of contentment or even happiness. Indeed, we are now seeing increasing numbers of older people going through the same relationship anxieties and stresses that we presumed only occurred in the young. Working in general practice can serve as a pertinent reminder that older people suffer the same fears and stresses as younger ones, but because they come from a generation that was taught to internalise their problems they might not feel comfortable talking about their worries, or seeking medical help.

Early in my career as a GP, I met Peter, a pleasant 85-year-old gentleman who was the sole carer for his 86-year-old wife who he had met over sixty years ago. Peter was of a generation that still approached visiting the doctor as being like any other professional meeting, and as such always dressed impeccably. In addition to being well turned out, Peter was also remarkably fit for his age, walked only with a cane (more for reassurance than actual support), still drove and he had a sharp wit and good mental acuity. He wore glasses, was always cleanly shaven, and had retained a full head of hair. But I rarely saw Peter for anything to do with his health. Peter's wife Mary had become increasingly frail over the last few years. Whereas Peter had retained all his faculties (both physical and mental), in contrast, Mary had become more and more absent-minded. Initially she forgot little things like where she had put her keys, or what day it was. But this gradually progressed to more significant problems such as forgetting to take her medication and her children's names. Throughout this decline in mental health and increasing fragility, Peter looked after his wife with no external help. He repeatedly declined the offer of carers, or any additional support, even from his own children. When Mary forgot that she was no longer working and attempted to take the car out (subsequently crashing it into the garage), Peter decided that he needed some help, and he brought his wife to see me to discuss finally getting a diagnosis and how we could move forward.

Mary had a full history and examination, memory and blood tests, and a CT scan of her brain. Each time I saw the couple, I would sit Peter and Mary down and reintroduce myself to Mary, who appeared to have no recollection of ever having met me before. I was not entirely convinced she even understood that she was at a doctor's surgery. We often discussed their problematic social situation, the difficulties with home life and how Peter was managing. But despite the demands of Mary increasing and Peter's own health beginning to fail, he continued to refuse any further input, insisting that as her husband it was his marital and lifelong duty to care for his wife for as long as he was physically and mentally able. Many times, Peter quoted at me, 'In sickness and health, Dr Foster.'

On receiving her test results, I brought Peter and Mary back to see me. Although the standard investigations (such as those for anaemia and diabetes) had come back normal, the combination of the scan of her brain and other more specific tests had confirmed a diagnosis of dementia. This in itself was not surprising, and Peter took the news well, probably suspecting this diagnosis for some time; however, dementia is an umbrella term, which encompasses a range of underlying causes from Alzheimer's disease to Parkinson's-related dementia, and Mary had been found to have an extremely rare cause for her condition. Mary had a disease known as 'general paresis' or neurosyphilis, and this was much harder for Peter to comprehend. I recall he looked understandably shocked at the diagnosis, and asked me to explain how this situation could have occurred and what it actually meant. I told him that neurosyphilis was a long-term complication of exposure to the sexually transmitted disease syphilis, usually from decades ago. The condition, if untreated, could remain hidden in the body for many years. Although it might have been difficult to discuss or recall, I asked Peter if there were any situations he was aware of that could explain how his wife might have contracted this disease, and also did we need to think about testing him too? To make an already difficult conversation worse, throughout our discussion, Mary sat inert, staring at her husband with a masked and emotionless expression, recognising her husband in some capacity but clearly with no sign of any understanding of the dialogue we were having.

Peter was understandably distressed and protested strongly that he had always been faithful and had never been away from his wife for more than three or four weeks since he fought in the Second World War. Peter briefly touched on the fact that he had suspected his wife might have had an affair early in their relationship while he had been fighting abroad but that this had never been confirmed. After the war, Peter returned to England as a veteran, but he had considerable difficulty adapting to civilian life. He said he was often withdrawn, found himself very anxious in social situations and was plagued with nightmares and flashbacks. With modern awareness, Peter would have been diagnosed as having post-traumatic stress disorder, but there was no such recognition of this condition at that time. Over many years of self-reflection and difficulty, Peter learned to manage his condition, but it consequently meant that difficult topics, such as a possible affair, were never discussed.

Peter's expression was a strange combination of anger and almost bereavement. 'What do I do now?' he asked me. I explained that Mary would need to be referred to a specialist clinic for review, as her condition was very rare. I felt that the possibility of any real improvement, however, was doubtful. But this was not the answer to the question Peter was really asking me. 'How do I care for a woman who has kept this secret for the last 50 years and now expects me to look after her when she's like this?' he continued. Peter's frustration had reached a point of being almost tearful and he struggled with what to say next. I tried to fill the gap, and explained that it was still his wife sitting next to him, and no matter what had happened in the past, she had obviously loved him as they had stayed together for more than 50 years. Peter looked at his wife and then me and replied despondently, 'But I can't even ask her.' To this, I had no answer, but could only offer my support.

After what felt like minutes, Peter thanked me (as always), got up and ushered his wife to follow him out. For the first time he did not say goodbye, but walked slowly and solemnly out of my office. Mary obediently followed her husband, gave me a broad smile and said goodbye to me in a happy demeanour, depressingly oblivious to her husband's distress.

Anticipating that Peter and Mary's home situation was likely to become more fractious over the next few weeks, our practice made great efforts to try to support the couple. In addition to Mary being referred to the hospital specialist, we contacted Age UK, MIND, the local psychiatry team and social services in an effort to try to provide as much help as we could. Our senior nurse, who helped manage our complex patients, was in regular contact with all the external agencies involved, and she and I also made great efforts to touch base with Peter regularly to check if he was coping. But despite the influx of additional support, over the subsequent weeks I saw Peter and Mary less and less.

Several months passed, and work and holidays got in the way. Eventually, when less distracted, I made a concerted effort to reach out to the couple to check on their well-being, but I found that they had left the practice. Perhaps because I felt guilty for leaving it so long, I contacted Mary's son, who informed me that she had gone into a nursing home only a few weeks after their last appointment with me. Peter had been diagnosed with depression and was now on medication. He had moved down south to be closer to his children and grandchildren. It turned out that the nursing home where Mary now lived was only a few miles from our practice, and with the permission of the family, I called the home for an update on Mary, to find out that her health had declined, she was reclusive and rarely had any visitors. The carers had met her children on a few occasions, but no one else ever came to visit. I was really more curious about Peter, but the carer said that she had never actually met him. For all intents and purposes, Mary, who had previously had decades of a loving and close relationship, appeared to be alone as she reached the end of her life. Hearing that Mary had now been deserted added to my sense of guilt, as I felt responsible for delivering the life-changing diagnosis to the couple, which inadvertently had contributed to their relationship breakdown.

As GPs, we see hundreds of patients every week, and it is our ability to compartmentalise and reset ourselves every ten minutes that allows us to function effectively. Each patient is greeted by a fresh, 'Hello, how may I help you today?' irrespective of the emotional burden the previous patient might have brought us. Over time, GPs become increasingly immune to these stresses – it is our method of coping; however, we all have certain patients that stay with us. Often, these patients are the ones we feel that we have failed, but they also remind us of why we became doctors in the first place.

CHAPTER 4

Erectile dysfunction

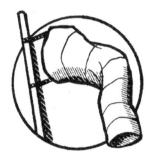

T he understandable stigma that surrounds erectile dysfunction (ED) means that it is one of the most difficult
problems for men to talk about. As a result, by the time
that most men have decided to speak to a doctor they have
already suffered with ED for months or even years and they
will have already made extensive Internet research, and
might have even tried legal or illegal therapies in a desperate
attempt to avoid having that embarrassing conversation. It
is also true that many doctors shy away from the topic of
ED, also finding it awkward and uncomfortable. The overall result means that it is common for those experiencing
ED to feel isolated and alone in their suffering.

In reality, the opposite is true and it is now well established that the global prevalence of ED is high. The Massachusetts Male Aging Study, performed between 1987 and 1989, was the first large-scale survey looking at the prevalence of ED, and found that over half of men aged 40–70 years had some form of erectile problem.[1] If ED is so common, then, why is it not talked about more openly, and managed better?

ED has been around since the dawn of man, and it affects men of all ages. But the very nature of ED, and its association with the intimate and personal topic of sex, means that it still remains a difficult conversation for patients and doctors alike. It is this aspect of ED that makes what is essentially a relatively straightforward medical problem into something we procrastinate about, trivialise and often ignore at our peril. Despite ED being around for thousands of years and affecting millions of men, we still treat it as if it is something to be sniggered at or ignored so as not to risk humiliation or embarrassment. All the while, if addressed properly, ED can usually be treated simply and effectively. But this only happens if a man is able to talk openly about the issue and is not left to simply buy a little blue pill.

Who gets erectile dysfunction?

We tend to associate ED with advancing age, because as we get older we are more likely to develop other medical problems that link to a decline in erectile function (these will be discussed in detail later). Younger men suffering with ED tend to have a greater psychological component as their cause, but it is important to stress that, in practice, there is usually a degree of both physical and psychological problems mixed together. This is because once a physical illness results in decreased erection quality, it commonly results in a profoundly negative association with sex, which can make it even harder to gain a normal erection in the future.

Unlike in the 20th century, men are now actively encouraged to talk openly about their problems, and ED should be no different. But not only do men still find it hard to speak to their doctor about it, but it can be just as difficult, if not more so, for men to talk about ED with their partner. A significant number of patients I see tell me that their relationships have actually been made worse by trying to discuss their erectile difficulties with their loved one. This pressure to perform, coupled with the anxiety of a partner who feels that they are no longer desired, can make ED worse and ultimately results in mental-health problems and/or the end of the relationship. This is why not only is it important to understand what causes ED but also that it has a major psychological component. By treating ED we are not just trying to improve a physiological process, we are also trying to improve a man's mental health and his attitude and approach towards sex.

What really causes erectile dysfunction?

The ability to produce an erection is a far more intricate activity than we might first suspect, involving a complex interaction between neurological, hormonal and vascular processes. We need a good blood supply to the penis, with healthy arteries and veins, a minimum level of testosterone and other hormones and a responsive neurological connection, as well as healthy skin and muscle. And on top of all this, we need to have desire. It is unsurprising therefore, that the causes of ED are so broad that many are often overlooked. In general, we classify the causes of ED as being either physical, psychological or a mixture of both.

Myth buster: true or false?

Myth: if you suffer with ED, it means that you are not attracted to your partner.

False. There are an enormous number of medical problems that cause erectile dysfunction, so having a partner who is sympathetic to the fact that it can be due to a medical problem and is not necessarily a reflection on the relationship, can significantly reduce stress and pressure for the patient.

There are so many different causes of ED that they can be split into different subgroups. These include: vascular causes affecting the blood vessels; neurological problems affecting the sensation or brain signals that trigger arousal; hormonal causes that suppress testosterone; and specific conditions that might directly affect the anatomy or function of the penis. Here are the most common problems in each area:

The most common problems that cause erectile dysfunction			
Vascular causes	Neurological causes	Hormonal causes	Individual causes
Cardiovascular disease	Parkinson's disease	Low testosterone	Trauma
High blood pressure	Stroke	High prolactin	Complications of surgery
Diabetes	Multiple sclerosis	Thyroid disease	Complications of radiotherapy
High cholesterol	Brain injury	Adrenal disease	Cancer
Smoking	Spinal cord disease		Anatomical problems (Peyronie's disease, congenital deformities)

Although the causes of ED are clearly broad, the most common physical cause is diabetes.[2] This is because poorly controlled diabetes affects so many of the processes required to achieve an erection, namely vascular, neurological and hormonal pathways. Cardiovascular disease is the second biggest physiological cause of ED and, in fact, the lining of the penile arteries and coronary arteries are so similar that they are both affected in the same way by cardiovascular risk factors such as obesity and smoking.

In addition to lifestyle factors, diabetes and cardiovascular contributors to ED, the other significant physiological cause of ED is low testosterone. Although not surprising, men who lack testosterone have problems with desire and also the ability to gain and maintain an erection.

In addition to the diseases and medical problems that can cause ED, it is common for a wide range of prescribed medicines, over-the-counter treatments and recreational drugs to contribute to the problem. The list below illustrates some of the more common medicines and drugs that have been linked to developing ED.

Antidepressants
Some blood pressure medicines
Antipsychotics
Anti-inflammatory steroids (prednisolone)
Opiates (such as codeine or morphine)
Anti-fungals
Certain antacid medicines
Cocaine
Heroin
Cannabis
Methadone
Anabolic steroid use
Alcohol
Some cancer therapies

Most of us do not read the leaflets inside our medicine packets or think seriously about the ways recreational drugs might affect our bodies when we use them. Therefore, if you suffer with ED, it is important to question whether something you are taking could be causing the problem and, where possible, could this drug be reduced, changed or even stopped? The effect of drug-induced ED is perhaps best illustrated in men suffering with depression, who might already struggle with a low libido due to their illness, which is then combined with an antidepressant treatment that actually worsens their erectile function and causes problems with ejaculation. This is, of course, not to advocate that antidepressants should not be used for fear of inducing sexual dysfunction, but rather that the doctor–patient conversation should allow this potential problem to be discussed and the correct medicine prescribed as a result.

'But I can just buy treatments for erectile dysfunction, so why see a doctor?'

The ability to buy over-the-counter treatments for ED is not new, but with the recent addition of Viagra now being available without prescription, it is easier than ever to avoid seeing a doctor about ED. But is this a good thing?

Many companies selling easy-access ED treatments actively promote the avoidance of having to see a doctor as a positive thing because it eliminates the awkward conversation. But, as mentioned above, there are a wide variety of causes of ED, and simply buying a tablet to improve erectile quality is treating the symptom without knowing or addressing the cause. At best, buying over-the-counter treatments helps reduce the psychological element of performance anxiety, but at worst it delays someone presenting to their doctor with a potentially serious medical problem because they were able to get symptomatic relief without a prescription.

Different treatments for ED are discussed in detail below, but my best advice is not to trivialise the symptoms. Before settling for any form of medication, make sure you know what has caused the ED in the first place, and ideally treat that as well. When looking at how to treat ED properly, it is important to consider the following three areas:

1. Always aim to find and treat the underlying cause.
2. Use appropriate medication to help improve function.
3. Address any psychological or relationship issues.

The little blue pill

Almost everyone has heard of Viagra and knows what it is for. Millions of men take it worldwide, and it has revolutionised the treatment of ED. Prior to Viagra, management of ED was very difficult for patients and doctors alike, with treatment options being limited to either injections directly into the penis, external devices such as vacuum pumps, or even surgery. With the advent of Viagra, which was patented in 1996, came an affordable, non-invasive and easy-to-take medicine that could be given to patients in the community, and it was extremely successful; however, despite its global success, Viagra was actually discovered by accident. Pfizer (the company who manufacture Viagra) were actually trying to develop a new drug for high blood pressure and heart disease and found that while the cardio-vascular benefits of the drug were limited the unintended erection benefits were significant. As a consequence, the intended purpose of the drug was changed, and with it the way we globally approach the treatment of ED.

Viagra comes from a group of drugs called phospho-diesterase type 5 (PDE5) inhibitors, which work by increasing blood flow to the penis when it is needed. It is important to stress that this increase in blood flow is not constant during the time the pill is in the body. Unless you are sexually aroused, Viagra should not give you an erection. Since the introduction of Viagra, there have been several other PDE5 inhibitors developed, all with different benefits, intended actions and side effects. This means that it is now possible to take an ED medicine that has few side effects, fits a patient's lifestyle and helps to put back some of the spontaneity that is part of romance. Some of the most common PDE5 inhibitors used in the treatment of ED are included in the table on page 150.

One of the most common problems with ED treatments is matching patient expectations with what the treatments can actually achieve and finding the right medication for the individual. It is important to stress that other side effects are also recognised when using PDE5 inhibitors, and there are some pre-existing medical problems that mean that they cannot be used by everyone. But this is part of the reason why it is so important to discuss these treatments with an appropriate health professional.

In November 2017 it became legal for Viagra to be sold without prescription in the UK. It was anticipated that for many thousands of men this would help to reduce the anxiety of having to see their doctor to discuss ED issues or

Common PDE5 inhibitors

Drug	Also known as	Speed of onset	Duration of action	Main reason to use	Common side effects
Sildenafil	Viagra, Viagra-Connect, Revatio	30–60 minutes	4–6 hours	First choice treatment for many with ED. It's been around the longest, and has the largest evidence base	Visual disturbance, headaches, and occasional nasal congestion
Tadalafil	Cialis, Adcirca, Tadacip	20–30 minutes	24–36 hours	Longer lasting, means it can be used without having to worry about spontaneity	Generally same as Viagra but can be longer lasting
Vardenafil	Levitra, Staxyn, Vivanza	10 minutes	5–7 hours	Rapid onset so it can be used for those wanting an immediate effect	Not to be used in patients with abnormal heart rhythms
Avanafil	Stendra	30–45 minutes	5 hours	Limited data at present but considered to be fast-acting	Limited data at present as only been out since 2012 and is not yet commonly prescribed

source the pills illegally online; however, this has actually had an unintended negative consequence for the general health of men. As discussed above, there are a variety of serious and non-serious medical problems that can result in ED, therefore the single most important aspect of treating the condition is working out why it developed in the first place. Being able to access treatment over the counter removes that initial conversation with a doctor and puts patients at greater risk of missing an earlier diagnosis. Therefore, the unintended consequence of over-the-counter Viagra has meant that men might wait longer to see their doctors, usually when the Viagra has stopped working, or when whatever underlying medical problem causing their ED has become worse.

Second- and third-line therapies for ED

Of course, Viagra is not effective, desired or tolerated by every man who suffers with ED, and other treatments, although used less often, do exist. The only other physical treatments for ED that do not require a prescription are the vacuum-erection devices, which although preceding the discovery of Viagra still remain a viable alternative treatment for some men. Common side effects include bruising, local pain and failure to ejaculate, and partners also report that the penis often feels cold. Overall, despite its relative success rate, vacuum devices are now not commonly used as a treatment for ED.

Other prescription medicines for treatment of ED include the use of drugs that cause dilation of the penile blood vessels through the action of prostaglandins. These drugs are effectively the gold-standard test for erectile function, as their mechanism of action causes a localised dilating effect that means an erection will occur even without any neurological stimulus (or desire). The downside to these medications is that they are given either via an injection into the base of the penis or as a cream that goes into the urethra at the tip. Where these medicines are either not suitable, or fail to work, surgical treatments include penile prosthetics (implants surgically inserted into the penis), which can be either malleable or inflatable. Understandably, they are used in only a small proportion of patients due to the low number of cases that require this procedure, plus the success it provides is limited.

Finally, it is worth noting the recent introduction of extra-corporeal shock wave therapy (ESWT) for ED. ESWT is a non-surgical treatment (similar to ultrasound) that works by delivering impulses of energy targeted to specific tissues, which increase blood flow and stimulate cell regeneration and healing, and can remove the need for medication altogether in some patients. ESWT has been widely used in various other forms of musculoskeletal injuries, and although still in its infancy with respect to ED treatment, the evidence for its use is promising.

Addressing the psychology

Sometimes, when looking at treating ED, we put a disproportionately heavy emphasis on medical therapies and neglect the psychological element that inevitably accompanies the condition; for example, at a basic level, the key question that all men should be asking themselves before they are resigned to a diagnosis of ED is whether they actually want to have sex with their partner? Desire, performance anxiety, premature ejaculation or the negative cycle that ED itself can create, unsurprisingly makes medical treatment even more challenging.

In patients where there is likely to be a significant psychological element, getting appropriate psychosexual counselling is crucial. This might be in the form of couples counselling, individual therapy to address any underlying psychological trauma, or something specific to sex itself. It is also worth noting that psychosexual counselling is a specialist form of therapy and is not something that would be easily treated by non-specialist-trained counsellors or therapists.

Summary

- Over half of all men will suffer with some form of erectile dysfunction at some point in their lives.
- Despite how common it is, ED remains a difficult topic to discuss with partners, friends and even doctors. As such, it can negatively affect the mental health of patients and impact on their relationships.
- There are a large number of medical causes of ED, and most patients have some element of psychological overlap that understandably accompanies the condition.

→

- Modern treatments for ED are highly effective in most cases, but they rely on addressing and treating the underlying cause.
- Over-the-counter treatments for ED remove the chance to get to discuss the problem with a doctor and can lead to serious illnesses being missed.
- In addition to Viagra, there is a range of other specific, highly effective ED treatments.

ED is more common that you might think, but if you are suffering with it, my advice is to speak to a doctor now. By addressing the problem early it will save you time, money and anxiety – and could even save your life.

CASE STUDY

The cheater

Matt was brought in by two paramedics who rushed him into the emergency department with a sense of panic and urgency that one rarely sees outside cardiac arrests or TV dramas. Matt was obviously extremely distressed, his shouting and screaming being audible throughout the department. Even the paramedics that had brought him in appeared anxious. But except for the screams of agony and a large sheet tented over his groin, Matt appeared to be physically well. The senior nurse attempted to measure his observations including his temperature, pulse and blood pressure, and his numbers all read normal, but clearly something very bad had happened.

Matt was in his early forties, with thinning hair and the wrinkled face of someone who spent little time smiling. While he continued to flounder and curse, the nurse began drawing up some morphine to relieve his pain, and I attempted to find out what had brought Matt into hospital. His response was brief and succinct:

'What's happened?!' he said in a rather condescending and irate tone. 'I'll tell you what happened. I've snapped my fucking penis!'

Even after nearly 20 years in medicine, this is still not a common response to the opening question of, 'What has brought you in today?', so once we had suitably calmed Matt, and reduced his pain, I persuaded him to expand on his opening statement.

Matt had been married for 15 years to a woman a year younger than him and who, in his words, 'did a shitload of exercise'. According to Matt, she was obsessed, and this obsession had grown over the last few years to the point where she had now developed an athletic and muscular physique. Sadly for Matt this had become quite a turn-off, as it turned out that he had a penchant for larger women. In fact, the disparity between how his wife now looked and Matt's underlying sexual desires had led him to start having an affair with a woman twice his weight and half his age.

The affair had been going on for several years, and Matt's wife had been completely oblivious to his adultery throughout this time, blaming his lack of sexual desire on the classic downward spiral of middle age. From Matt's perspective, he spent long hours at work and had become more overweight. He used to nap in the evenings and displayed little or no sexual desire towards her. For all intents and purposes, Matt had become the poster boy for low testosterone, appearing to be an unmotivated, non-energetic, desexualised, 40-something-year-old man. In reality however, Matt had been having lots of sex – just not with his wife.

On the day of Matt's admission to hospital, he had met his mistress at her home for lunch. Unsurprisingly, just as with previous working lunches, one thing had led to another, and they ended up going upstairs for dessert. The exact nature of what happened next made every male doctor or nurse who heard this story wince and recoil in revulsion. During their lovemaking, Matt's mistress had been on top, and due to her incredible size, it made normal sex difficult. Matt explained that as she rose above him, she had come up too far, his penis exited her vagina, and she then came down with the full weight of her twenty-stone body onto his erect shaft. The result was a sudden 'popping' sound, rapid bruising and the appearance of what is termed 'the eggplant penis', as the shaft swells and rapidly fills with blood. In addition, there was a lot of pain.

While mild cases of penile injury can be treated with ice packs or anti-inflammatories, Matt needed to see a surgeon, and quickly, as the injury had occurred over three hours ago and there was a good chance that this might end up with either a permanent deformity of his penis, or even amputation.

As the urological surgeon discussed the operation with Matt, I assisted in documentation, pain relief and blood taking, before asking him if there was anyone he wanted me to contact to explain where he was. Matt was clear in his response:

'Don't you dare tell my wife!' he said aggressively.

'Then what should I say if she rings to ask where you are?' I replied.

'I don't know,' he responded again rudely, 'just make up some shit.'

With that closing comment, Matt was wheeled away by theatre staff and could be heard swearing and abusing them as they took him out of the department and down the long corridor towards the operating theatres. Even as he turned the corner out of sight, he was still heard shouting:

'You hear me?! Don't tell my wife!'

As if by comedic irony, about ten minutes later, I was told by the nurse in charge that I had a phone call from Matt's wife who wanted to know what had happened to her husband. Clearly, I could not go against the express wishes of the patient, but I felt I could not avoid the question completely as it would be obvious something was wrong when she next saw him with surgical bandages over his groin. Therefore, as requested by Matt, I conjured up my best attempt at improvisation, and promptly failed miserably.

'Your husband has had an injury to his penis,' I explained, realising that this was not a good start at avoiding the topic.

'Unfortunately, while erect it came into contact with a large solid object, which caused impact at high speed, and which has resulted in him needing an emergency operation.'

I waited for the reply, and for a moment I thought I might have got away with it, but Matt's wife had only paused, and then she asked me 'Was it a car accident? I don't quite understand.'

'No,' I replied steadily, and realised that I had now reached the limit of my improvisation skills, and needed to get out of this situation quickly. 'No. The rest of him has not been injured,' I carried on. 'Just his penis. I am sure he would appreciate seeing . . . ' But before I could continue, Matt's wife interrupted me.

'But you say he came into contact with a large object? What sort of object?' she asked more forcefully, clearly concerned that I was not being totally transparent with her. Now really starting to panic I felt I had to terminate the conversation as fast as possible, so cleverly, I replied:

'All I can say is that the object was large enough to break his penis, but has not harmed anything else and he has not brought it with him.'

At this point I looked up in sheer panic, desperate to receive some support from the senior nurse standing next to me, but on looking at her all I could see was that she appeared to be crying, tears of laughter streaming down her face, as she gripped her sides and tried maintain her composure. I carried on: 'He's in theatre now, but I'm sure he'd love to see you after. He's on the urology ward.' And before she could ask me anything else, I hung up, made my excuses and decided I needed to go for my break immediately.

I did not meet Matt again, and never spoke again to his wife, but I was informed that she did not come to visit him in hospital. Post-surgery, Matt spent a week on the ward, the operation had not gone particularly well, and the time delay in getting him to theatre, combined with the force of the trauma, had meant that part of his penis had been amputated. I was told by a friend of mine who worked on the surgical ward that throughout his hospital stay, Matt had received no visitors, and on the day of his discharge, no one came to help him to his taxi. In the end, Matt left the hospital alone, a very different man from the one that came in.

CHAPTER 5

Baldness

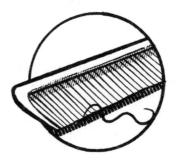

G rowing up in the 1980s and 1990s, I remember several of my secondary-school teachers who struggled with hair loss, growing the hair on one side of their head much longer than the other, and pulling the long side across their scalp, so as to provide the illusion of a full head of hair. This was the infamous comb-over. Understandably, it fooled no one, and the already obvious attempt to hide their receding hair was made worse by any sudden gust of wind, which would inevitably lift the hair away from the head. Worse than that, as naïve teenagers, we openly mocked these attempts at disguise. But with the benefit of age and experience, it is easy to see why so many men felt that they had no choice but to go to such lengths to maintain the illusion of a full head of hair.

Since the 1980s, the world has become even more image obsessed. The media continues to impress on us what it defines as beautiful, but now social media, airbrushing and appearance manipulation apps further add to our feelings of inadequacy and anxiety over our own body image. It is unsurprising then that men worry that going bald is more than just a simple cosmetic problem to be shrugged off or trivialised.

Although the world has changed since the 1980s, our DNA has not. Four out of five men will still suffer some degree of hair loss as they get older, and for some men, this process can begin as early as their teens. How we manage this problem varies from person to person, but as treatments have advanced, some men are willing to go to extreme measures to try to avoid losing their hair.

What is baldness really?

There are many different types of hair loss, with causes ranging from stress, localised fungal infections and nutritional deficiencies to hormonal problems. But the most common form of hair loss is androgenic alopecia, also known as male-pattern baldness. Despite its name, androgenic alopecia is a genetic condition that actually affects both men and women. This means that if we are going to go bald, the decision is made when we are in the womb. We tend to think of baldness as the progressive loss of hair, but in reality, androgenic alopecia is actually the gradual conversion of terminal hairs (the thick hair we usually have on our heads) to vellus hair (the barely noticeable and extremely fine hair we see in baldness). Interestingly, the vellus hair of a bald person is the same type of hair we see on the bodies of young children, which tends to be softer and finer. As puberty begins, these hairs change to terminal hairs and become thicker, longer and more apparent.

Why some hair recedes and then appears to halt mid-head whereas others continue to go on to complete baldness is unknown, but the largest contributing factor remains genetics. Interestingly, there has been a link proposed between male-pattern baldness and an enlarged prostate gland,[1] as well possible links between baldness and the development of kidney stones.[2] But what is the process behind androgenic alopecia that actually results in hair loss?

Myth buster: true or false?

Myth: being bald means that I have more testosterone.

False. Baldness is not related to how much testosterone you have. But it *is* a measure of how sensitive you are to it.

It is often rumoured that bald men have higher levels of testosterone than their full-headed counterparts, and while the majority of people dismiss this as nonsense, it is not completely untrue. In certain parts of the body, testosterone is converted to another, more active male sex hormone, dihydrotestosterone (DHT). In essence, DHT is just a very potent form of testosterone. It has a similar role to its parent hormone and is essential for the development of our second-ary sexual characteristics during puberty (such as pubic hair and maturation of the penis and scrotum) as well as being responsible for enlarging the prostate gland as we get older (this is covered in more detail in Chapter 8). It is also DHT that is the main cause of hair loss. An enzyme known as 5-alpha reductase is responsible for the conversion of testos-terone to DHT, and it is found mainly in the prostate gland, the skin and the hair follicles. Patients with more 5-alpha reductase enzymes, or hair follicles more sensitive to DHT, will end up going bald. Therefore, having no testosterone will prevent hair loss, but having more testosterone does not mean baldness is inevitable.

Overall, age, stress and many other factors contribute to hair loss. But genes play the biggest role, and the best predictor to gauge if you will go bald is simply to look at the other men in your family.

Why are men so worried about their hair?

For those of us lucky enough to still have our hair, it can be difficult to appreciate just how devastating it can be for those who have lost theirs, particularly in early adulthood. Hair is associated with youth, virility and attractiveness, and it is a major component of our body image. We grow up seeing ourselves in the mirror daily, learning to accept and under-stand the reflection we see back as our own. We can all recall how distressed we have been after having a bad haircut. Now imagine there is no hair at all, and the process is irreversible.

Baldness is clearly more than just a cosmetic issue. It can be associated with low self-esteem, depression and a loss of confidence. We can all name a handful of famous bald actors, but the ratio of hairy to hairless A-list celebrities is not even close to representing the general population. Western society still places great value on a youthful appearance and hair loss is seen as a step away from the Hollywood ideal.

Admittedly, not all men worry about going bald, and some are able to face the challenge of hair loss with little or no concern. But this is about individual confidence and the ability to accept changes in our body as we age. Luckily, fashion and culture has evolved and when men do start to go bald, they can now shave their heads and retain an image of social acceptance and attractiveness. We no longer have to accept the bald spot as the inevitable product of thinning male hair. Indeed, some men with no hair loss at all choose to shave their heads completely to promote a persona of increased masculinity. However, this only applies to those men that have a choice. We all have to make adjustments in our lives and amend our expectations as we get older, and our approach towards baldness should be no different.

What if I don't want to go bald?

For those unwilling, or unable, to accept going bald, hair-loss treatments have improved so much over the last 40 years that for the majority of men it is now possible to slow down, halt or even reverse the hair-loss process. The biggest problem that most men face when deciding on hair-restoration products is the fact that the market is so large, and it can be a daunting task working out which treatments are effective and which are useless gimmicks. The hair-loss industry is massive, worth more than £1.5 billion globally per year. A quick Internet search for baldness treatment reveals an enormous range of options including foams, sprays, vitamins, lasers, scalp massagers, collagen stimulators and surgery. It is, therefore, understandable that a man who is anxious about losing his hair might try several different products in the desperate hope that it will restore his hair.

In practice, treatment for baldness is relatively simple. This is because there are only a handful of treatments that are actually proven to work and are safe for people to use. It is probably worth noting at this point that there might be other effective and legitimate hair-loss treatments available, but this book is only concerned with those products that have been proven to be effective, safe and evidence-based. I have avoided mentioning any treatments that have not been licensed for hair loss or with success claims made only by the individual product or a handful of customers advocating, 'It worked for me, and it can work for you too.'

Licensed treatments for male-pattern baldness fall into two main categories: surgical, and non-surgical. Non-surgical treatments are generally oral medicines or topical treatments, and they tend to be a less risky and cheaper option (in the short term). The biggest problem with non-surgical treatments is the impermanent nature of their mechanism: if you stop using the drug, the baldness comes back. Surgical hair restoration is now a highly specialist and effective procedure for most men; however, even with these factors in mind, the initial cost and risks associated with surgical procedures still mean that for most men medical therapies remain the initial choice in hair-loss treatment.

Medical treatments

There are a range of medicines and alternative therapies that claim to help to restore hair loss; however, it is important to be aware that many of these treatments have no evidence to back up their claims and may not be safe. Non-evidence-based treatments include hair oils, collagen stimulators, beer, Tabasco or even bull semen. In fact, when it comes to non-surgical treatment of baldness, there are only two medications that are licensed for use: minoxidil and finasteride. No other medications, creams or lotions have been shown to be as effective, and there is no merit in using other forms of treatment that are unlikely to yield any significantly positive results.

Minoxidil

A topical treatment for hair loss, minoxidil is available as either a spray or a foam. It is very effective, and patients tend to notice positive regrowth of hair within about three months. Amazingly, no one really knows how minoxidil works. It was originally invented to treat blood pressure but was found to have the side effects of increased hair growth.

Although usually well tolerated, a common side effect of minoxidil is skin irritation. Alternative preparations might resolve this problem, or switching to a different form of treatment (such as changing from using the foam to using the spray). The biggest problem with minoxidil is that it has to be applied twice a day, and to avoid hair loss returning, it will need to be used forever.

Finasteride

Finasteride is as a once-a-day tablet and is primarily a drug used to shrink large prostate glands. It acts by preventing the conversion of testosterone to the more active DHT, which, as discussed earlier, is linked to the development of hair loss.

Finasteride has been shown to be very effective in slowing and even reversing hair loss, but because it is taken orally, patients are also subject to the other side effects. These effects include: erectile dysfunction, ejaculation problems, decreased libido and even gynaecomastia (male breasts).

Effective treatment can take up to two years. Just as for any other medical treatment for hair loss, once the treatment is stopped, the hair loss returns.

Surgical treatment

The principle of surgical hair restoration is to take hair from a more densely populated area of hair growth (usually the back of the head) and literally transplant it to the thinner area. Surgical hair-restoration therapy really came into practice in the late 1980s and at that time the standard procedure was to take large grafts – that is, plugs of 10 to 20 hairs – and implant them in clumps. Obviously, the final results were variable. Since then, the technology and techniques around hair transplantation have been significantly advanced and refined.

In general, there are two types of hair-transplantation surgery: follicular unit transplantation (FUT), and follicular unit extraction (FUE). FUT is an older procedure, which involves taking a strip of hairy skin from the back of the head and inserting the hair into another area of the scalp. FUE is more refined, and involves removing hair follicles directly from the scalp for transplantation to other areas. In both procedures, modern technology now allows for individual hair follicles to be transplanted, and the final results are much more natural in appearance.

Hair transplant procedures usually take between four and eight hours, depending on the amount of hair required to transplant or the complexity of the procedure, and the surgery is usually done all in one sitting under local anaesthetic. Which operation is most appropriate is determined on a case-by-case basis, but the risks of surgery remain broadly the same for both types of procedure. These include bleeding, infection, scarring or failure of the operation. The biggest factor that usually stops men opting for surgical hair restoration, however, is the cost, which can be anywhere from a few thousand pounds to more than £30,000.

Baldness affects some men in such a profound way that it can have a deep psychological impact on their mental health. Seeing the lengths that some men will go to in an attempt to conceal their hair loss is astounding, but we do not have to suffer in the way that my teachers did in the 1980s and 1990s. Modern treatments have provided a range of successful and safe options for preventing and reversing hair loss, and it now means that men have far greater choice in how they manage their appearance. With new cosmetic technologies being developed all the time, perhaps the bigger challenge we will face in the future is how we learn to accept our own bodies, rather than trying to change ourselves to meet the perceived expectations of society.

Summary

- By the age of 50, more than three-quarters of men will have significantly thinner hair.
- Despite its prevalence, hair loss can cause significant anxiety and distress.
- Bald men do not necessarily have more testosterone, but they are more sensitive to its more potent derivative, dihydrotestosterone.
- There are many effective treatments for male-pattern baldness. These include:

Minoxidil A topical treatment applied twice a day that is available as either a foam or spray and has been shown to improve hair growth significantly in balding men.

Finasteride A once-a-day tablet, which has been shown to significantly improve hair restoration for men with thinning hair.

Hair transplant surgery Now a highly precise and effective procedure, but which is often costly.

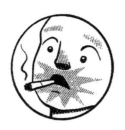

CASE STUDY

Paul the puffer

The first thing that hit me as I walked into the resus area of A&E was the smell of smoke, cigarettes, and the overwhelming stench of burnt hair. For anyone who hasn't smelt burnt hair, it has a quite distinctive odour, owing to the fact that human hair contains keratin, which, when set alight, releases some of its sulphur-containing properties. At the centre of the aroma was a skinny, red-faced man with no eyebrows, half his hair missing and a lot of wet bandages covering the rest of his scalp and head.

It was immediately obvious that the patient, Paul, was struggling to breathe, and due to the fact that he had been involved in some form of fire-related accident, our first priority was to make sure his airways and lungs were safe. After some time treating Paul it appeared, in fact, that most of his symptoms were due to panic, and as his condition improved, I took the opportunity to find out how he had ended up in hospital.

Paul suffered with emphysema: a form of lung disease commonly brought on by smoking. He had become addicted to cigarettes at the age of 15, and during most of his thirties and forties he had smoked more than 30 cigarettes a day. Although he had now reduced this number, Paul told me that his main reason for cutting down had not been illness but what he described as 'the extortionate rise in the cost of cigarettes. But that was then, doc,' he went on, 'I only smoke 15 or so a day now, and most of them are roll-ups.' I tried to explain that roll-ups were probably worse for him, as the filter was even less protective, but I felt that this was perhaps not the best time to start lecturing a man who had just lost his eyebrows.

In addition to the various inhalers and medicines that Paul needed for his chest condition, in recent years his lungs had become so damaged that he now required home oxygen. It was administered through a small tube inserted into each nostril and, on further discussion, Paul confessed that he probably relied on the oxygen so much that he would leave the tubes on his face all day.

When using home oxygen it is important to remember to keep any naked flames at least six feet away, due to the potential risk of explosion. Paul had made it clear to me that he was usually very good at this, always remembering to turn off his oxygen tank, and giving time for the oxygen to disperse into the air, while he rolled up his cigarette. Sadly, for some unknown reason on this day, Paul had forgotten his own routine, and although he had popped the nasal tubes out of his nose, he had left them on his face with the oxygen still flowing.

'I'm not sure why I did that,' he protested, 'it must have been while I was watching *Homes under the Hammer.*'

Consequently, as Paul lit his match and brought the naked flame towards his mouth, a jet of fire shot up his face, obliterating his eyebrows, most of the hair on his head and crisping a significant amount of skin, too. Amazingly, he avoided any damage to his eyes and sustained no other serious injuries.

Paul had always maintained a good head of hair, and he found its loss a particularly distressing aspect of his trauma. Once he was aware that his lungs were not damaged (any further), Paul became fixated on his head, worried that his hair would never recover or grow back to what it was. As bizarre as this seemed, while smoking had aged, damaged and disfigured him, Paul's hair had remained a constant, meaning that when he saw his reflection in the mirror, it still bore a likeness to the person he used to be 20 years ago. For Paul, his hair was more than cosmetic. It was a link to a time before the walking frame, oxygen tanks and disability.

Doctors are trained to make decisions in the best interests of their patients, and this can make it easy for us to become arrogant, believing that we know what is best for the patient. I recall many of my colleagues, myself included, holding back from castigating Paul for not appreciating how lucky he was to be alive. After realising how close he had been to death, how could he not be more grateful for all we had done for him?

Shortly after Paul had been reviewed by the plastic surgeons, he was transferred out of the department and I never saw him again. One of the problems with working in emergency medicine is that you rarely find out what happens to your patients once they leave the department. Often one is left to speculate at their recovery, how they manage on the ward, undergo rehabilitation, and how difficult it might be to make that journey home as a different person. This was certainly the case with Paul, as even if his hair did grow back, it was going to take many months, something I was sure he was going to struggle with emotionally. Although physically his injuries were not severe, appearing even comical in nature, the psychological impact of Paul's accident had been devastating: the loss of his hair taking away the last part of his former identity, and robbing him of a meaningful piece of who he used to be.

CHAPTER 6

To Beard or Not to Beard

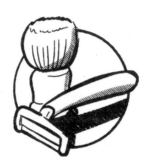

As with many aspects of fashion, trends tend to rotate in cycles, and the popularity of beards is no different. In the last few years, there has been a resurgence of men displaying facial hair, and this is reflected in the number of beard grooming products that are now available. But beards are not like flared trousers or tank tops; there is something intrinsically masculine about the presence of a full and well-groomed beard on a man. Although the social and cosmetic relevance of beards might vary from decade to decade, there is no doubt that the presence of a beard provides its owner with a sense of gravitas and authority, which can help boost confidence and self-esteem. In fact, as beards have become more fashionable once again, the desire to grow facial hair has become so important for some men that the inability to do so can lead to a form of beard anxiety. Although heavily influenced by our genes, it is important to be aware that there are medical problems that can significantly affect beard growth, and by identifying these issues, in many cases hair growth can be restored, or at least improved.

Why do we have beards?

Beards are arguably the most visible sign that an adolescent male has reached maturity and is theoretically able to father a child. From a physiological perspective, one cannot grow a beard without sufficient levels of testosterone to stimulate the facial hair follicles into action. But as we have already seen, nothing in medicine is simple, and more testosterone does not automatically result in a hairier face.

In a similar way that the hair on our heads is affected by testosterone, beard hair follows a similar (although not identical) pattern. As we saw in the last chapter, around 10 per cent of the testosterone in our blood is converted to a more potent testosterone by-product called dihydrotestosterone (DHT). Although testosterone prepares the hair follicles for growth, it is the DHT, activated by the enzymes in the oil gland of the hair follicles, that is responsible for the growth of facial hair. On average, a fully developed beard grows just over a centimetre per month.

It is understood that men with high levels of DHT and a greater sensitivity to the hormone will be able to grow beards at a younger age than other less productive or sensitive men. As discussed in the previous chapter, it is this same hormone (DHT) that is not only responsible for beard growth but is also responsible for male-pattern baldness. This is why, on average, bald men are often able to grow a good-quality beard. But is this development of facial hair an evolutionary relic from our primitive ancestors, or does it continue to serve a useful function, especially in today's modern world?

It is extremely unlikely that beards have evolved as a random fluke of evolution, as nature only permits the progression of a developmental trait that adds some advantage to our chances of either reproducing or survival. It is often assumed that men with beards are perceived as more attractive to women than their hairless counterparts. But in reality, there is little evidence to support this, and studies are contradictory in how attractive bearded men are actually rated. Certainly, this inconsistency in results suggests that the primary function of a beard is not to secure a mate.

It has been suggested that as cavemen the presence of facial hair acted as a display of masculinity and power. The beard was intended to act as a show of dominance and seniority towards other men, and to help impose a position as the alpha male in the group. Interestingly, some of these traits have persisted in modern society. Even now, men with beards are perceived as older, stronger and more aggressive than those who are clean-shaven. Although we might not need to worry about evolutionary advantages, these benefits can still provide modern men with additional confidence and a feeling of empowerment that could improve the chances of success in various aspects of life.

The causes of poor beard growth

Poor beard growth can be divided into two main areas: failure to ever grow any substantial facial hair, and secondary loss of an existing beard that was previously well established.

In terms of primary beard growth, this is usually determined by a series of factors we have little or no control over, such as genetics, age and ethnicity. As we age, our bodies become more receptive to DHT, which means that it is invariably easier to grow a beard when we are 40 years old than when we are 20. Ethnicity also plays an important factor when looking at facial hair growth, with men from a Mediterranean background commonly being hairier than those of East Asian descent.

One factor that might be alterable is testosterone, as this is required for conversion to DHT and the subsequent stimulation of facial hair; however, it is only in patients with significant testosterone deficiency that hair loss or absence would be present, and it would also be expected to be associated with a variety of other problems.

Although the mechanism that results in facial hair growth is different from that which produces the hair on our heads, there is some crossover with systemic illnesses that can affect both; for example, significant malnutrition, autoimmune disease or chemotherapies will produce a global loss of hair, but not only will this be apparent in the widespread hair loss that results but it will also tend to be accompanied by other medical symptoms or signs.

When it comes to secondary facial hair loss, the causes

tend to be easier to treat, and they usually result in a patchy appearance rather than the complete loss of hair. One of the most common causes of patchy hair loss is due to a fungal infection in the skin known as ringworm. Thankfully, ringworm is not actually a worm, and its correct terminology is dermatophytosis. It has been nick-named 'ringworm' due to the fact that when the fungus affects the skin it results in an expanding worm-shaped ring. When it has an impact on beard growth, discrete areas or hair loss might be visible, often with an associated itch or dryness to the skin. Ringworm is a common condition and can often be treated successfully with antifungal medications within 2–4 weeks.

Alopecia barbae is an autoimmune condition where the body's own immune system attacks itself. Like ringworm, this can result in patchy hair loss, but often the underlying skin looks normal. The reason why some people develop *Alopecia barbae* is not fully understand, but it is seen more commonly in those with other autoimmune conditions such as type-1 diabetes and lupus, and also in acute forms of stress. Treatment for this condition is far more difficult, with no definitive cure being available, which means that most sufferers require the input of a dermatologist.

It is worth also highlighting that extreme changes in lifestyle can also result in patchy or global facial hair loss. Examples include prolonged stress (although this is also likely due to a suppression in testosterone), major dietary changes or restrictions, and even over-grooming of the beard; for example, although using a boar-bristle beard brush can benefit a beard in terms of removing debris and keeping it looking good, brushing too aggressively and too often might cause damage and thinning of the hair. Even washing beards too frequently can result in the formation of brittle or damaged hair and irritation of the underlying skin layer.

The challenge of shaving

At first glance, this might seem a rather trivial problem, as after all shaving is basically just cutting hair. But, unlike a haircut, which is designed to trim or sculpt hair into a specific length or style, the challenge of shaving is to cut the beard hair as short as possible without harming the skin beneath. Men have been shaving for thousands of years, and it remains the most common cosmetic ritual that men perform. But even though the tools we use to shave with have advanced and become more sophisticated, the complications of shaving and skin reactions that often occur remain a constant challenge for shaver manufacturers.

Shaving has been around for so long that it is surprising that we have still not yet been able to invent a single device that allows us to cut our facial hair down to the skin layer but does not carry the risk of discomfort, bleeding or irritation of the skin. Wet shaves still require multiple strokes, they have to be performed in a certain direction, and they can result in dryness or irritant reactions to the skin or might cause bleeding. The reason for this is that beard hair grows in a different way from the hair on our heads, and the skin on our faces is particularly sensitive.

Compared with the rest of our bodies, beard hair is often more dense, thicker and stiff, and it has an acute emerging angle (meaning that it protrudes from the skin at an angle that is more difficult to cut), and it grows more quickly. To make matters worse, the skin on our faces is more sensitive than most of the rest of our body, so it is not unreasonable that the repeated scraping of our faces with a sharp blade would result in skin problems.

Myth buster: true or false?

Myth: shaving makes facial hair grow back thicker.

False. Hair thickness has nothing to do with how often it is cut. By the time a hair strand is at the surface of the skin it is dead, which means that follicular diameter and the density of hair cannot be altered by trimming or shaving.

Beard anxiety

Society dictates that we should be manly. This means acting tough, looking tough and suppressing our emotions. Despite various attempts to encourage men to fight against this pressure, especially when it comes to mental health and discussing our emotions, how we are expected to look has not really followed this trend. We are living in an odd period in male culture where we are encouraged to tell people how we feel, discuss our emotions and even cry when necessary, but we are also still expected to look tough and masculine. And nothing epitomises the look of toughness and masculinity as a full beard.

The problem is that while beards are now back in fashion, and it is almost expected that we should be able to grow one simply by desire alone, it has become increasingly obvious that for many men, growing the facial hair they wish to achieve is not always possible. It is this inability to grow any significant facial hair that can cause frustration, worry and even a degree of anxiety, and can lead to feelings of inadequacy and being less masculine compared with those who can achieve a full beard.

The anxiety and frustration that can accompany the inability to grow facial hair is a relatively new phenomenon driven largely by social and cultural pressures that did not exist in previous periods in history. How we look and present ourselves today is constantly evaluated and critiqued in a way that simply did not happen the last time beards were in fashion in the 1970s. For younger men, it can be deeply upsetting socialising with their bearded friends who appear more confident and charismatic, while their own baby-faced appearance means that they get ID'd trying to buy a round of drinks. A few years ago, one of my patients, aged 22, who was particularly troubled by his lack of facial hair, said to me, 'Who would you trust to save your life? Harry Potter or Dumbledore?' It is this desperation to keep up with social expectations that drives many men to buy products from the beard-grooming industry in the hope that it will result in a better-quality beard.

What can you do to improve the growth of your beard?

Before going any further into what might or might not contribute to beard growth, it is important to note that the primary determining factor that decides how well we can develop our facial hair is genetics. It is worth looking at your father, grandfather or older brother as a good predictor of what you might be able to achieve in the future, but even this is only an estimate. Our potential for beard growth is determined by the number and density of our hair follicles, our sensitivity to the hormone DHT and how much DHT is circulating in our system. There are other mitigating factors such as malnutrition or medical problems that might affect hair growth, but in a fit and healthy man, the number of hair follicles, DHT, and follicle sensitivity are the three core variables that determine our degree of facial hair growth, and they are all largely decided by our genes.

Once we understand how much is out of our control when it comes to facial hair, it allows us to focus on what can actually be done and avoid spending precious time and money on gimmicks or novelty solutions that are never going to work.

Testosterone

When it comes to beard growth, the first myth to dispel is the concept that more testosterone will automatically result in a better beard. As we have established above, it is not the total amount of testosterone that influences our facial hair, but the proportion of DHT, as well as how sensitive our hair follicles are to this hormone. It is correct in assuming that if you were significantly testosterone deficient, normalising your testosterone levels would result in a greater proportion of active DHT, and this would help to grow facial hair, but the converse is not true. Super-dosing on testosterone might result in more of it being converted to DHT, and this will undoubtedly have some effect on increasing hair growth. But sensitivity to the hormone remains the same, and once the hair follicles are saturated there is little more that can be achieved. All the DHT in the world will not cause new hair follicles to grow where they were not genetically programmed to do so. In addition, taking very high levels of testosterone is dangerous.

Exercise

It has been proposed that by increasing our exercise we can improve blood flow to the face and therefore help with hair follicle stimulation. Exercise can also stimulate testosterone production. The theory of this sounds reasonable, but in fact not only is there no evidence to back this up but also it makes little sense from a physiological perspective. If it was just a matter of warming up our faces to improve follicle activation, we could gain the same benefit in hair growth by sitting in front of a heater. There is no doubt that reducing the blood supply to a hair follicle will result in poorer hair growth, but assuming the opposite must also be true, and that by warming our faces up through exercise will in some way stimulate beard growth, does not really make sense.

Furthermore, when it comes to testosterone, only about 10 per cent is converted to DHT, and the testosterone spurt we gain from exercise is unlikely to result in any significant prolonged change in circulating levels of DHT.

Diet

We have already established that good nutrition obtained from eating a healthy, balanced diet is crucial for all aspects of our health. And just like any other body part, facial hair needs proper nutrients to establish and maintain normal growth. It is therefore likely that dietary deficiencies or obesity will result in a decrease in our facial hair production or quality. In particular, the absence of basic vitamins such as vitamins A, B, C and E, and the mineral zinc, are likely to result in poorer hair quality. As a significant proportion of our hair is made up of protein, particularly restricting diets or those low in protein are also likely to affect hair development.

In addition to under-nutrition, obesity is also likely to result in a reduction in effective beard growth: obesity decreases the circulating levels of testosterone and, subsequently, DHT. (For more about diet and exercise see Chapter 2.)

Beard oils

Beard oils are generally used to groom and care for existing hair, but some products also claim to stimulate or improve development of new facial hair. The theory behind how this could work is multifactorial, but basically it relies on the massaging effect on the skin. It is claimed that by rubbing beard oils into the skin this helps to remove unwanted dead skin cells and other bits of debris that could have an impact on normal follicular growth. Other proposed benefits of beard oils include improved blood flow, help in controlling oil excesses in the skin and preventing bacteria proliferation. There is even some suggestion that certain oils might improve the strength and elasticity of the beard hair, making it appear thicker and less patchy.

Sadly, almost all these claims are without quality evidence to back them up, and at best these products offer small, unproven benefits, while at worst they are mere placebos. It is also worth considering what these claims mean in practice, and how much change to our facial hair we can reasonably expect to gain from massaging oil. Humans have evolved to produce the correct amount of natural oil required for our skin. We already have a very effective blood supply in our faces, and if we are concerned about debris or bacteria, we can always have a wash. There is no doubt that beard oils will effectively contribute to the cosmetic appearance, and even possibly the durability and quality of existing facial hair, but the difference they could have in stimulating new hair growth is negligible.

Derma rollers

Beard rollers, or derma rollers, are small, circular devices covered in tiny needles. The device is designed to be rolled over the face where the desired hair is to grow. The proposed mechanism behind how derma rollers work is actually simple:

1. The small needles of the beard roller puncture the skin in multiple places.
2. This causes micro-trauma and sets up an inflammatory reaction at each puncture source.
3. The inflammatory process leads to an increased localised blood supply and vessel dilation.
4. The improved blood supply and healing process causes increased nutrient and hormone absorption, resulting in better hair growth.

Of all the possible ways to improve beard growth, this appears to be the most bizarre, and users often find that areas of their face appear bloody or sore after using the device. Yet despite this, there does appear to be some evidence that this procedure could actually improve hair growth. Unsurprisingly, studies looking at the specific effects of derma rollers and beard growth are very limited, but the evidence we do have is encouraging.

Minoxidil

Primarily used in the treatment of male-pattern baldness, where it has been proven to be very effective (as we saw in Chapter 5), there has been some interest in the use of minoxidil to improve and encourage beard growth. Although studies have been very few, there is some limited data that suggests topical minoxidil does improve hair growth on faces as well as heads; however, what is not clear is whether minoxidil can stimulate *new* hair follicles to be active, or if the *existing* hair becomes thicker. It is also important to stress that minoxidil is primarily licensed for hair restoration on the head, and not on the face, and the sensitivity of facial skin can mean that users are more prone to its side effects. Overall though, minoxidil is a safe drug that can be bought without a prescription.

Beard transplant surgery

Recent advances in hair transplant surgery have resulted in a high-quality procedure that results in good outcomes for many men. It is not surprising, therefore, that beard transplant surgery has also started to become more popular.

The procedure is similar to hair transplant surgery, and it involves transplanting an area of good and stable hair growth (usually at the back of the head or behind the ears) onto the face. The procedure can take between three and nine hours to complete and is usually dependent on the transplant area required; for example, a moustache might need 1,000–1,500 hairs, while a full beard might need 4,000 hairs. Costs are highly variable and can be from a few thousand pounds to over £10,000.

Finally, and most importantly, do not obsess over something that is out of your control. When it comes to beards, our ability to achieve our desired appearance is largely determined by genetics. A small percentage of men might be able to find and treat an underlying cause for their scanty hair growth, but for the vast majority of us, our beard-growing potential is something predetermined before we were born. By learning to accept who we are it can make us happier in the long run, rather than chasing an ideal image of someone we feel we ought to be.

Summary

- How well we are able to grow a beard is principally determined by our genes.
- Products or concepts that will do little for the growth of your beard include:

  1 Taking extra vitamins or minerals
  2 Using beard oils
  3 Exercise

- Proven methods to improve beard growth:

  1 Make sure you have a balanced diet
  2 Avoid stress where possible
  3 Maintain a healthy weight
  4 Make sure you do not have low testosterone (by consulting with your doctor)

- If it is patchy or there is new hair loss, see a doctor, as there might be an underlying medical cause.
- Consider using minoxidil.
- Consider using derma rollers.
- Consider beard transplant surgery.

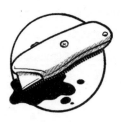

CASE STUDY

The curious case of Will, testicles and a Stanley knife

One evening a few years ago, I was the only doctor covering the minor injuries unit in a quiet cottage hospital. A very distressed nurse approached me and asked if I would assess a patient who had suffered an injury that she did not know how to manage. This was my first job as a senior doctor in emergency medicine. As a result, I was a little arrogant and self-assured, and patronisingly I replied to her, 'Of course I'll take a look. There's nothing I haven't seen before.'

On arrival at the bedside, I greeted Will, a 58-year-old, obese, grey-haired man who was naked from the waist down, apart from a blanket hiding his modesty. He smiled awkwardly, and while the nurse stood next to me, I introduced myself. 'Hi, I'm Dr Foster,' I said smugly, 'shall we take a look at the problem?' The nurse pulled back Will's blanket to reveal a normal penis and below, what looked like the end of a broccoli stump once the florets had been cut off. Looking more closely, the whole area where the scrotum should sit had been replaced by a distorted, bloody and gangrenous stump, held together by a ring of elastic bands. At this point, with my arrogance completely lost, I spluttered in a high-pitched tone, 'Where are your balls?'

To which Will, appearing completely relaxed, simply stated, 'I got rid of them.'

Will worked in banking, lived alone and coincidently suffered with Parkinson's disease. He also enjoyed drinking alcohol, which he would do regularly, and in large amounts. By drinking alcohol, Will found that this relaxed his tremor and allowed him to entertain his pastime of pleasuring himself while wrapping rubber bands around his scrotum.

As he lived alone, Will explained that he had been indulging in this practice for several years, but, over time, he had required more and tighter rubber bands to get the same degree of satisfaction. One eventful evening, Will had followed his usual routine of drinking alcohol and applying his rubber bands before entertaining himself; however, on this occasion, Will had consumed too much alcohol and had subsequently fallen asleep. For whatever reason, he had forgotten to remove the elastic bands the next day, and he only realised that something was wrong when he noticed an unpleasant odour emanating from his groin. At this stage, Will explained, quite calmly and rationally, that he then went out and purchased a Stanley knife and proceeded to cut off the dead tissue, which in practice meant his entire scrotum and testicles.

Up to this point, I hadn't really said anything, but seeing that Will had finished his story, I felt compelled to ask out of curiosity, 'So, where are your balls now?' Will replied dismissively, 'Oh, yeah sure. I flushed them down the loo. I mean, I don't need them any more?'

'What about kids?' I replied astonished. 'Or testosterone?' Will appeared to think for a moment, and then calmly replied, 'Oh yeah . . . I didn't think of that.'

Once I had had some time to compose myself and process what had just been discussed, I had to complete my assessment and treatment of Will. It turns out that the rubber bands he had applied to his scrotum were acting as a form of tourniquet, not only preventing him bleeding to death, but also preventing the infection from his necrotic and pus-filled stump tracking up into his body.

It was agreed that Will would need to be transferred to a specialist urological unit at the main hospital nearby. Luckily for me, my friend was the doctor on call for urology and accepting referrals, so I proceeded to page him and explain the reason for the transfer of care. Surgical on-calls can get very busy, and clearly when I spoke to my friend he was already swamped and in no mood for my call; however, his response was not what I expected.

'Bloody hell, Jeff!' he replied angrily. 'You know how busy I am, and you ring me making up bullshit about cut-off testicles. This isn't funny you know. I have better stuff to do than listen to your crappy humour. Just do your own work and stop messing around.' He then hung up on me.

Despite his reply, I took this to mean the transfer was agreed, and proceeded to send Will to the urology unit, advising the ambulance transport crew that he had been 'accepted with some reluctance'; however, 30 minutes later, I had a call back from my friend in urology.

'Oh God! I've just seen it!' he said apologetically. 'It's in my head now. I can't get it out of my mind! I thought you were just winding me up. My boss is coming in from home now, as I don't think he believes me either. This guy is gonna need a whole lot of work doing. We are prepping him for theatre now. Sorry for hanging up on you earlier, but it just didn't sound real. I'll keep you posted about what we do with him . . . Jesus, it's in my eyes!'

A few weeks later I did have a call from my urology colleague who informed me that not only had Will had several operations to get rid of the dead and infected tissue, but he had also remained in hospital having antibiotic treatment and been assessed for some prosthetic testicles. He was also going to need lifelong testosterone replacement therapy, and he was currently being assessed by psychiatry with a view to transfer to the psychiatric unit once stable. I was also informed that up to this point, it still remained unclear as to whether Will had been mentally ill when he amputated his own scrotum, as his explanation, although distressing, appeared quite logical. Either way, there were no immediate plans to allow him home.

CHAPTER 7

Everything You Ever Wanted to Know About Testicles

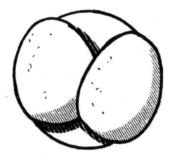

Our testicles are essential for two things: they produce testosterone and sperm. It therefore seems odd that from an evolutionary perspective, our most important organ required for us to reproduce lies exposed and dangles defencelessly at the front our bodies. Without testicles we would never go through puberty and develop all the features that make us men. Neither would we produce sperm. Yet despite the obvious importance of this organ, in many respects our testicles remain our Achilles heel, protected by nothing more than a flimsy scrotal bag and muscle that tries to pull them up when threatened.

Even from an early age, boys become aware of their testicles, and as we progress through life we become more conscious of their presence, their function and also their disease risk. Rarely, however, do we ask why we have evolved in such a way, and what the implications for our health and wellness are. This chapter is designed to help men understand more about one of our most unusual but crucial anatomical features, dispel some of the myths around our testicles and help us to understand how to check and monitor them for illness and disease.

What do testicles do?

Testicles, or testes, are oval-shaped organs that weigh about 10–15 grams each and hang in the scrotum, which supports them and helps to regulate their temperature. Other than a single muscle, the cremaster, which serves to try to pull the testicles up into the pelvis when we are attacked, they have little by way of protection and remain constantly exposed. Inside the scrotum each testicle is attached to a nerve, artery and vein, as well as the epididymis: a tube-like structure that acts to store and mature sperm so that it can fertilise an egg when necessary.

The human testes produce around 200 million sperm a day, but the reason why we (and so many other animals) have developed external genitalia, while others such as elephants and rhinoceroses have retained internal gonads, remains a mystery. We know that the primary reason for our testicles to be external is that sperm is best produced and stored at around 34 degrees centigrade, that is 2–3 degrees below normal body temperature. At body temperature, sperm become more active and mobile, but this is short-lived and only lasts for around one hour. This is just the right amount of time it takes for a sperm to reach a female egg after sexual activity. After a longer period than that, or at any higher temperature, the sperm become inactive and useless. Although this might explain how the process of human reproduction works, it does not explain why some animals have kept their testicles internal and still retained their fertility. One theory for development of external testicles is that the benefit of producing more effective and efficient sperm by lowering their temperature is worth the risk of keeping them exposed. In reality, however, these are just theories, the definitive reason for our exposed testicles is unknown.

Myth buster: true or false?

Myth: getting kicked in the groin hurts so much because our scrotum is part of our abdomen.

True. Getting a testicular injury not only causes us pain because our testicles are so poorly protected, but also many of the tissues that make up the scrotum are embryologically derived from our abdomen. As we develop, they descend into the scrotum. That's why getting hit in the groin makes us feel sick.

What can go wrong?

There are various disorders that can affect the testicles, the earliest of which can originate while we are developing in the womb. One rare condition, known as androgen insensitivity syndrome, is a genetic illness that results in a male foetus being unable to respond to the testosterone required to make it develop as a male. These babies are born with genitals that appear female, or between male and female, but a womb and ovaries don't develop internally, because genetically they are still male. Complete androgen insensitivity is a rare condition that affects only 2–5 births in 100,000. Much more common, however, is the problem of undescended testicles. As a male foetus develops, the testicles begin in the abdomen, and as the foetus grows, they are embryologically pulled down into the scrotum, so that by the time a baby is born, both testicles should have made their way into their correct final place. Undescended testicles are so common that one in 25 boys are born with at least one testicle that has not descended properly. This does not usually require treatment, as most will move to the correct position naturally over the next six months. Only around 1 per cent of boys will end up needing to have this problem surgically corrected.

Later on in life, other problems that can occur with our testicles include twisting or trapping on their stalk (torsion), infections, blocked tubes or even cancer. But serious testicular problems remain rare, and most common ailments just tend to cause testicular discomfort or swelling, or mild pain. The list below highlights the most common disorders that you are likely to come across:

Epididymitis

The epididymis is a long, coiled tube that stores sperm and transports it from the testes through the male reproductive tract. Epididymitis is inflammation or infection of the epididymis and it can be caused by sexually transmitted diseases, injury – or from no obvious cause at all. The symptoms of epididymitis might include pain (from mild to severe), swelling of the testicles or scrotum, nausea and vomiting, and fever. It is one of the most common testicular disorders, it is not serious and it is usually treated with antibiotics.

Hydrocele

A hydrocele is a collection of fluid that forms around the testicles. It is a generally painless fluid swelling in the scrotum, but it can be uncomfortable depending on the underlying cause, such as an infection, the beginnings of a hernia (where an internal part of the body pushes through a weakness in the muscle or surrounding tissue wall, in this case, into the scrotum), or even cancer. Hydroceles do not always have to be treated, but it is important to scan them to find out why they have formed.

Varicocele

A varicocele is like having varicose veins in the testicles. Just like a hydrocele, it is generally painless, but it is said to feel like a 'bag of worms', in the scrotum. Varicoceles are generally considered harmless, but once there they will not resolve by themselves, as just like a varicose vein anywhere else in the body, the damaged veins cannot be repaired without surgical intervention. It is important to stress that although they do not have to be treated, if large enough, the increased blood supply might warm up the testicle affected and decrease sperm production and fertility.

Spermatocele

Often also known as a spermatic cyst, these fluid-filled sacs are often easy to feel on self-examination, and they are the leading reason that men will present to their doctor worried that they might have testicular cancer. In practice, although spermatoceles might be worrisome as they present as hard lumps and can lead to discomfort or pain, they are not sinister and usually do not need treatment.

Orchitis

Orchitis is inflammation of one or both testicles. In general, orchitis is caused by infection, the most common being sexually transmitted diseases such as chlamydia or gonorrhoea. Orchitis can also be caused by mumps. Worryingly, the anti-vaccine movement has resulted in an increased number of younger men, and even children, presenting to emergency departments with acute orchitis due to mumps from failing to vaccinate. Sadly, this can have a catastrophic effect on future fertility.

Torsion

As mentioned above, testicular torsion occurs when the spermatic cord gets twisted and cuts off the blood supply to the testicle. Although this is rare, it is a medical emergency that requires immediate surgery in order to save the testicle. Symptoms include the sudden onset of severe pain with possible swelling and tenderness of the testicles and scrotum. Patients might also notice fever, nausea and vomiting. In such cases the best action is to seek medical advice urgently.

The 'C' word

Men worry about getting testicular cancer more than almost any other malignancy, and yet it only has an incidence of around 2,400 new cases in the UK per year. This makes it the seventeenth most common cancer in men, accounting for only 1 per cent of all male cancers. But it is the connotations of what testicular cancer means for us that promotes such vivid fear and worry. Interestingly, over the last ten years, the incidence of testicular cancer has increased by almost a tenth, but this is unlikely to be due to changes in prevalence of the disease, and more likely due to a greater awareness of the condition by doctors and patients. If you are unlucky enough to get testicular cancer, survival rates are very good, with an average 98 per cent survival rate at ten years.

Unlike the more common cancers (such as bowel cancer or lung cancer), testicular cancer is not affected by known carcinogens such as smoking or alcohol. As such, reducing the risk of testicular cancer through lifestyle is very difficult. There is little evidence that being overweight or exercising alters our risk of the disease, and nor does stress or what we eat. But we do know that children identified as having undescended testes should be surgically corrected as soon as possible as this can increase future cancer risk, and there have also been some studies that have suggested that women exposed to certain chemicals during pregnancy could increase the risk of their future male offspring being either infertile or developing testicular cancer. This is not really a modifiable risk factor though, as an adult male can do nothing about what his mother did while he was in her womb. Overall, there are no proven ways to reduce the risk of getting testicular cancer through lifestyle modification. Therefore, we rely on recognising the symptoms and checking ourselves for changes or abnormal lumps. The symptoms of testicular cancer include:

- A lump in the testicle (the most common symptom, appearing in over 95 per cent of cases), which is usually painless, but does not have to be.
- Testicular pain.
- A dragging sensation in the scrotum.
- Hydrocele, which presents as painless fluid that accumulates and causes the scrotum to swell. As explained on page 196, although most are benign, you should always get it checked.
- Male breasts (gynaecomastia) due to release of a hormone called beta-human chorionic gonadotrophin (beta-hCG), which is produced in larger amounts in testicular cancer.

Self-examination

There are no blood or urine screening tests that we can
do effectively to check for testicular cancer, and over the
last few decades doctors and male-health advocates have
developed and promoted the concept of self-examination.
Self-examination refers to each man literally feeling their
own testicles on a regular basis to systematically check for
lumps or abnormal growths. Although testicular cancer
is rare, self-examination helps us to understand what is
normal for our testicles, and it might also help us to diagnose some of the problems listed above. In general, most
men have one testicle larger than the other and one also
tends to sit higher in the scrotum. It is common to be able
to feel small cysts that sit in the epididymis, but these tend
to be rubbery in nature, mobile and not directly fixed to
the testicles. I would recommend self-examining your testicles once a month and using a systematic approach, as
illustrated below.

Common sense would suggest that self-examination is an
obvious and easy way for us to check ourselves for testicular cancer, but does it really make a difference? One of the
earliest recorded suggestions that performing testicular self-
examination would be a way to help improve the chance
of finding disease dates back to 1977 in a medical article
entitled 'Various ways in which individuals can help detect
cancers early'. Unlike modern medicine where everything
we do is backed up by evidence, safety and proven effectiveness (or as close as we can get), in the 1970s the same rules
did not apply. The concept of self-examination was quickly
adopted by men and doctors alike, as it felt like a quick,

Self-examination for testicular cancer

1) Check your testicles at least once a month

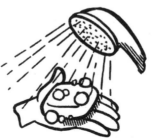

2) Perform your check in the shower with soapy hands

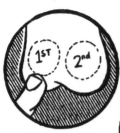

3) Check one testicle at a time

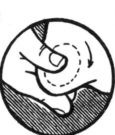

4) Gently roll each testicle between your finger and thumb

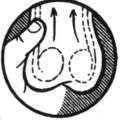

5) Feel along the spermatic cords at the back of the testicles

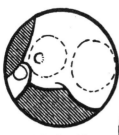

6) Look for hard lumps or rounded bumps

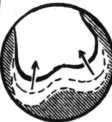

7) Check for changes in size and shape

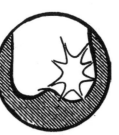

8) Check for any painful areas

non-invasive and relatively simple process to perform. It is still widely promoted today, despite the fact that the pick-up rate for cancer through testicular examination is so low that it would take 50,000 men examining themselves for 10 years to prevent one death from testicular cancer.

This, however, is not really the point of self-examination, and it does not mean that you should not do it. Many male cancers such as prostate cancer as well as testicular cancer have no screening process or tests available, and there are virtually no modifiable risk factors, especially for testicular cancer. This means that whatever you do in your life, you are unlikely to be able to reduce the chances of getting testicular cancer. To compound the problem, funding for research into specific male cancers remains much lower than for female cancers. This is due to a variety of reasons including disease prevalence (breast cancer, for example, is far more common than testicular cancer), health implications, the severity of certain cancers, and media pressure and activity. Rather, the greatest benefit of self-examination of the testicles is to raise general awareness.

I have had heated exchanges with some doctors who feel that by promoting self-examination, we are likely to promote unnecessary anxiety in the majority of men who find a lump, as they will turn out to have nothing more than a benign cyst. But I have always countered this argument with the suggestion that I would rather instil a degree of anxiety for a number of men who are indeed healthy, if it ends up saving the life of another who otherwise might not have thought to check himself.

Looking after your testicles

When it comes to testicles, the take-home message is to look after them, but not to worry too much. Do self-examine, speak to a doctor if you are concerned or feel something is unusual, but do not become preoccupied over checking them or worry that something sinister will occur.

As objectively odd-looking as they might appear, our testicles are a major part of what makes us male, and in addition, their health and function is crucial to the very existence and evolution of the human race. By understanding the essentials of what our testicles do and what can go wrong, it allows us to better understand our bodies and helps us to take responsibility for our own health without obsessing about the things that don't matter.

Summary

- Our testicles are required to produce testosterone and sperm. Without them boys will not develop into men and will not be able to reproduce.
- Abnormalities in the scrotum are common, and include simple cysts, varicose veins and hernias.
- But serious conditions affecting the testicles, most importantly testicular cancer, are rare.
- The majority of treatments for testicular problems are effective, and even testicular cancer, when caught early, has a good outcome.

→

- There are no screening programmes available for testicular cancer.
- In addition, there are no lifestyle modifications that you can make to reduce your risk of testicular cancer.
- Despite its low pick-up rate, testicular self-examination remains the only method we have to check easily for abnormal lumps or growths in our scrotum.
- If you feel something abnormal on self-examination, get your doctor to check it, but do not worry – the vast majority of lumps turn out to be benign.
- Due to their fragility and the fundamental importance our testicles have in our lives, we disproportionately fixate on testicular health. But, thankfully, serious testicular disease remains rare.

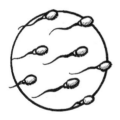

CASE STUDY

Love alone

There is a growing acceptance that just because we age this does not mean that we stop being sexually active. Historically, it was expected that once we hit our middle years we would lose our interest in sex, and certainly that by the time we retire it is only a distant memory. But with both men and women living longer, female HRT being more effective and testosterone replacement therapy (TRT) and Viagra in men being better accepted, it is quite natural that we might wish to remain sexually active in our senior years. Commonly, when the topic of sexual activity and ageing is discussed with my younger medical students, it is viewed with a combination of repulsion and curiosity. How could someone at 60, so old, want to have sex?

I was recently approached by a television producer who was trying to see if they could make a programme about sexually transmitted disease in the over-fifties. Marriage no longer means for life, and many people explore new relationships after their children have grown up, often forgetting the rules around safe sex because pregnancy might not be an issue. The concept was certainly very interesting, but in the end it was decided that so few senior patients would be willing to talk about their romantic and sexual problems on television that the idea was dropped. Nevertheless, we should not forget that just because someone does not suffer the emotional insecurities of teenage youth, they are still subject to the same joys, excitements and risks that come with dating and sex.

Tariq was 67, very overweight and a frequent attender at the practice. He always had some form of old food stain on his shirt, and he rarely saw the same doctor for more than a few appointments before choosing a new favourite a month or so later. When I saw Tariq, it was a hot June afternoon and he appeared flushed and uncomfortable as he entered my office.

'How can I help you today?' I asked. This is the opening line I use to greet all my patients.

'I want you to test if I can get an erection,' said Tariq quite bluntly.

'I'm sorry,' I asked, obviously hoping I had misheard. 'Could you elaborate a little?' I was hoping that there was more to this initial statement, otherwise this consultation was going to become uncomfortable very quickly.

'I want you to see if I can get an erection or not,' Tariq repeated, 'I need to know if it still works okay.'

'Why do you think that? Have you been sexually active recently? Perhaps you could give me a bit more detail about what's led you to this point?' I replied, again hoping that this was not the start of a conversation that ended up with me pressing the panic button on the wall. To be fair, sometimes I find that the awkward questions patients ask are actually due to simple embarrassment, and once they elaborate on their condition it is often the case that they suffer with underlying erectile dysfunction, performance anxiety or another medical or psychological problem that they have difficulty talking about.

'Yes, I am sexually active,' Tariq answered me again, without displaying any hint of emotion or embarrassment. 'I try as often as possible. I actually think that I injured myself the other week and that's really why I'm here. I need to know if there is a test you can do to make me have an erection.'

I politely explained to Tariq that, in reality, although specialist urology clinics can test for physiological erectile function, this was not possible to do in a GP surgery. I also clarified that for the average man an erection was not achievable unless accompanied by sexual desire. As I wasn't planning on my afternoon turning out that way, he agreed to drop the subject, and instead quickly turned his attention to a new topic, asking me:

'I try to be sexually active as much as I can but it hurts a lot if I do it too much, so I was also worried if I could be infertile.'

'Do you *mean* infertile?' I enquired. 'Are you thinking of having any more children?'

At this point, Tariq become slightly irate, replying with, 'I know what infertile means! No, I don't think I'm going to have any more children, but I wanted to know.'

'So, just to check, you are regularly sexually active now?' I wanted to clarify. 'Despite the pain?'

'*YES!*' Tariq appeared almost angry at the apparent ignorance of my question.

'With someone else?' I continued.

'No', he replied. 'Why does that matter?'

I knew Tariq was married; he had informed me that he was not having an affair and his sexual activity was entirely by himself. Over the next 20 minutes I tried to understand why he was so keen to know if he was still fertile, but there was no obvious reason. In the end, I put the idea to Tariq that he might be suffering with a form of health anxiety relating to his sexual function and suggested that treatment might be more beneficial from a psychological per-spective rather than just looking at physical function.

Health anxiety is an issue that we are seeing people struggle with more and more often in GP surgeries, and it is not uncommon for men to become fixated or anxious over the look and function of their genitalia. But successful treatment of this problem is extremely difficult, as it requires the patient to understand that their condition might be psychological rather than a physical problem. In reality, most patients leave the consultation feeling as if they have not been listened to. After all, 'How can it be in my head when the pain feels so real?'

Unsurprisingly, Tariq did not take my suggestion well, and did not come back to see me; however, I found out that two weeks later he had seen another male GP concerned over the volume of semen he produced, and a few weeks after that, he had made multiple appointments with a female GP colleague and had tried to show her his penis on every visit, worried that his ability to conceive had been impaired apparently due to some recent personal exploits.

CHAPTER 8

Prostate Health

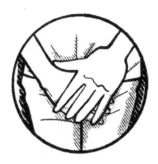

The prostate is an odd gland. It is something that all men talk about at some point in their lives. We know it causes problems for us as we get older, and we even see adverts advocating getting it checked when we stop to urinate at motorway services. But rarely do we appreciate what the prostate gland actually does, and why we become so obsessed with it as we age.

Only men have a prostate gland. Before puberty it is relatively dormant, but when activated by testosterone during adolescence it becomes an important organ for producing semen, as well as providing much of the force that occurs during ejaculation. The prostate sits just below the bladder and is usually about the size of a walnut, but one of the peculiarities of the gland is that, provided it is exposed to testosterone, it will keep growing as we get older. This means that it can end up being the size of a tennis ball, or even larger. It is this slow and progressive growth that causes problems for so many men, because although not being directly related to our kidneys or urine production, the prostate is intrinsically linked to our urinary flow, as the urethra (the tube we pee out of) runs right through the middle of the gland. Therefore, if the prostate gland gets bigger, and it invariably will as we age, this compresses the urethra, and our urinary flow weakens. Of course, the different medical problems that can affect the prostate might cause us to have additional symptoms, but almost all diseases that affect the prostate will alter urinary function in some way.

In general, there are only three things that commonly go wrong with the prostate:

1. It can become infected or inflamed (prostatitis).
2. It can grow too large (benign prostatic hyper-plasia, BPH).
3. It can become cancerous.

This should make diagnosing and treating any problems that arise in the prostate relatively straightforward, but medicine is rarely as simple as it should be, and the prostate gland is no exception.

Benign prostatic hyperplasia (BPH)

I recently went to a restaurant with my eight-year-old son, and when we both had to go to the toilet he took great delight in standing next to me at the urinal and passing urine with such force that he was able to direct a jet of fluid above his own head. After proceeding to mock me for my pitiful attempts at producing any comparable urinary force, it made me wonder at what age I lost the ability to pee with such precision.

There is no doubt that as we age our urinary flow decreases, commonly (but not always) due to the effects of prostate growth. But this is such a gradual process that we don't really notice it because we tend to lack any form of comparison. When we do go to a public toilet, we tend not to stand next to other men, assess their age and subsequently look to see how powerful their urinary flow is. As such, our own decline in pressure is something we really only take notice of when it starts to have an impact on our daily lives.

As the prostate grows bigger and compresses the urethra, it results in the classic urinary-tract symptoms we come to associate with getting older. The main symptoms of a large prostate include:

- Reduced urinary flow.
- Difficulty starting to pass urine (hesitancy).
- Increased urinary frequency.
- Urinary urgency (the loss of a gradual urge to go, but needing it suddenly instead).
- Waking up at night to go to the toilet.

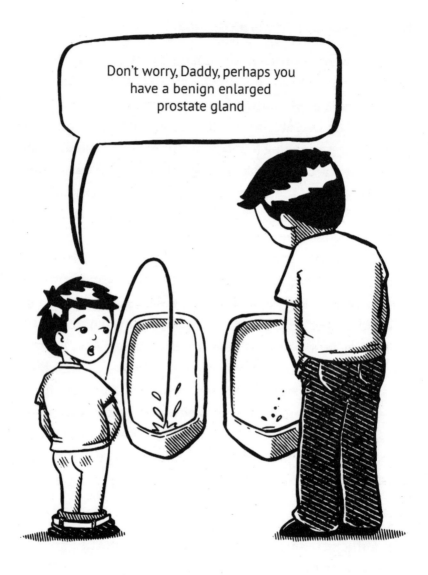

Around 50 per cent of men over the age of 60, and nearly 90 per cent of men in their nineties, have some symptoms of an enlarged prostate gland. These men would benefit from treatment because, in addition to the inconvenience a large prostate has on daily urinary function, a severely enlarged prostate gland can lead to urinary tract infections, bleeding, kidney disease and even acute retention (where one is completely unable to pass urine).

Medical treatments

Thankfully, the treatments for a non-cancerous large prostate (BPH) are highly effective and include both medical and surgical options. Medicines can be used to relax the smooth muscle in the prostate and bladder, which allows urine to flow more easily. Examples of this drug include tamsulosin (an alpha blocker), which in other forms can also be used to treat high blood pressure.

Other medicines used in the treatment of BPH work by blocking the stimulant effects of testosterone on the prostate gland. This effectively shrinks the prostate and improves symptoms. Examples of this type of medicine include finasteride, which, as we have seen, in smaller doses is used to treat baldness.

Just as with many medicines we use, it is important to stress that no treatment for BPH is without risk. Alpha blockers are generally well tolerated but can cause dry ejaculation (achieving orgasm without any semen being released). In addition, they do not alter the actual size of the prostate gland, and although they buy time for the patient, they do not stop the progressive growth of the prostate as it continues to compress the outflow tube. Finasteride, while highly effective in reducing prostate size, often has other side effects that come with suppressing part of the testosterone pathway. These side effects include erectile dysfunction, male breast tissue and a reduced ejaculation volume.

Natural treatments

In terms of natural medicines for treating BPH, there are more than 20 different products available. Most of these can be purchased from herbal and health-food shops, but sadly evidence for their safety and success is highly variable. Treatments include stinging-nettle root, soya, cranberry and prickly-pear cactus. Although most herbal medicines used in the treatment of BPH have little or no therapeutic benefit, there is good evidence that saw palmetto, a herb commonly sold as an effective treatment for big prostates, is not only ineffective but can actually be harmful. Overall, there are no herbal medicines that have been shown to reduce prostate size or slow disease progression; however, treatments such as African plum tree bark or rye pollen have been shown to help in easing symptoms, at least temporarily.

Surgery

When it comes to the medical and herbal treatments for BPH, there have been no new significant developments for many years. The same cannot be said for surgery. Historically, the most common surgical treatment for BPH has been a procedure known as a TURP (transurethral resection of the prostate). This involves a device called a resectoscope, which is a thin metal tube containing a light, a camera and a loop of wire. The tube is passed up through the penis into the urethra until it reaches the prostate, whereby the loop of wire is heated with an electric current and used to literally cut and bore away the section of prostate causing the symptoms. A thin tube called a catheter is then inserted to irrigate and pump fluid into the bladder to flush away the pieces of prostate that have been cut off.

As gruesome as this sounds, the TURP procedure has proven to be a highly effective procedure for millions of men worldwide; however, due to its invasive nature, it is associated with some risks, and post-surgical complications include bleeding, urinary retention, an inability to ejaculate properly, and even incontinence.

Recently, however, advances in technology have radically changed the way in which we treat BPH surgically, and there are now several options that are just as effective as a TURP, although considerably safer and more tolerable. These include the use of green-light lasers to cut the prostate (which reduces the risk of bleeding or infection), the uro-lift procedure (which literally lifts and holds the enlarged prostate out of the way), and even a steam treatment that requires no cutting of the prostate and is associated with very few complications.

Overall, having a non-cancerous but large prostate gland is something most of us will suffer with at some stage in our lives, but with treatments improving year on year, symptoms we historically accepted as just part of getting old are now something we do not have to endure.

Prostatitis

Prostatitis is basically just inflammation of the prostate. It can be due to a range of causes including bacterial infections, sexually transmitted diseases, immune problems including HIV, and, in some cases, no identifiable cause at all. Even relatively innocuous activities such as long-distance cycling can result in prostatitis due to the prolonged direct pressure on the perineum caused by bicycle saddles (cycling is also associated with perineal numbness and erectile dysfunction).

It is estimated that 15 per cent of all men will suffer with symptoms of prostatitis at some point in their lives,[1] and for most men symptoms will be uncomfortable but easily treated by their GP. Just as the symptoms of BPH commonly affect the urinary tract, the same is true for prostatitis; however, in addition to the effects on urinary function and flow, the key features of prostatitis are usually pain and feeling unwell. The other classic feature of prostatitis is how fast the symptoms come on. Although some cases of prostatitis can be long-standing, most are due to an acute inflammatory process, which means that there is often a sudden pain on passing urine, discomfort in the perineum (the area between the scrotum and rectum) or even flu-like symptoms.

Investigations for prostatitis include urine testing for infection, blood tests and sometimes scans of the pelvis. The prostate specific antigen PSA test (discussed in detail in 'Screening for prostate cancer' on page 221) is also usually raised, as it reflects the inflamed nature of the prostate. It is essential that if a PSA is used to aid in the diagnosis of prostatitis, it will be repeated after treatment to make sure that the level has returned to normal.

Obviously, effective treatment for prostatitis depends on the cause, but common therapies include antibiotics, anti-inflammatories or a referral to a specialist if the symptoms do not resolve. It is uncommon for prostatitis to be due to an underlying prostate cancer, but not impossible, and the condition highlights the complexities around PSA testing, which can be high in both an inflamed prostate and a cancerous one; however, for the vast majority of men, taking the appropriate antibiotic combined with removing the trigger, such as a catheter or practising safe sex, is enough to cure prostatitis.

Prostate cancer

Prostate cancer is the most common cancer in men in the UK and it accounts for over a quarter of all male cancer diagnoses.[2] The second most common cancers in men are lung cancer (13 per cent) and bowel cancer (13 per cent) with the three conditions combined being responsible for more than half of all new cases of cancer each year. Prostate cancer is now so common that one in six men will be diagnosed with it at some point in their lives.

Although risk factors include being overweight, having unsafe sex, alcohol consumption, being from an African-Caribbean background, or having other family members affected, the single biggest risk factor for developing prostate cancer is age. It is estimated that between the ages of

70 and 80 more than half of all men will have some micro-scopic evidence of prostate cancer[3] and it is plausible that were we to live long enough, virtually every man would develop malignant cells in their prostate gland.

In many ways prostate cancer is unique. This is because the presence of cancerous cells in the prostate does not automatically follow the decline in health that is usually associated with a cancer diagnosis in other organs. Unlike many other forms of cancer, which either grow rapidly or spread to other parts of the body (metastasise), the majority of prostate cancers remain localised to the pros-tate gland and develop at a very slow rate. This means that the risk of dying from the milder forms of prostate cancer, even if left untreated, is still only 7 per cent at 15 years follow up. In fact, the relatively slow growth of many forms of prostate cancer means that nearly half (45 per cent) of men diagnosed can undergo a process of watchful waiting, which means that they do not require active treatment, and they can simply be monitored by their specialist.

As we have established already, most conditions affecting the prostate gland tend to result in a change in urinary flow, so some of the common symptoms of prostate cancer are very similar to the ones for BPH (as described on page 211).

Unlike BPH, more advanced cases of prostate cancer might also have additional symptoms such as:

- Blood in the urine
- Blood in the semen
- Altered bowel symptoms

- Bone pain, usually in the pelvis, but potentially any-where in the body
- Impotence
- Enlarged lymph glands, usually in the pelvis area near to the prostate, but potentially in other regions of the body, too
- Weight loss and lethargy

If you are concerned that you might have prostate cancer, it is best to see your GP. In most cases your doctor will discuss the symptoms with you and is likely to examine your stomach and perform a digital rectal examination (this involves inserting a finger into the rectum to feel for any irregularities of the prostate gland) as well as performing a blood test, which looks for a raised level of prostate specific antigen (PSA) in particular. If there is a strong suspicion of cancer, you might also be referred for an MRI scan of the prostate to look for any abnormal areas within the gland. It is only then that a urologist would consider doing a biopsy to confirm a diagnosis.

When looking at treatment options for prostate cancer, it depends on the type of cancer diagnosed, how large or aggressive it is, and whether it has spread. In milder cases, watchful waiting or actively checking, but not necessar-ily treating the cancer, are common tools used to avoid unnecessary surgery. One might think that the mere diagno-sis of cancer means that it should be cut out or removed in whatever way is the most practical. Indeed, a Swedish study found that men with localised prostate cancer benefited from radical surgery to remove the prostate with a mean of 2.9

years of life gained.[4] In practice, however, radical surgery is not always the best option for a cancer that in many cases has a low mortality at 15 years even if nothing is done to treat it.

In cases where men are symptomatic, treatment options include complete surgical removal of the prostate (radical prostatectomy), radiotherapy, high-intensity ultrasound, drugs used to suppress testosterone and other forms of chemotherapy.

Overall, 77.6 per cent of men will be alive for more than 10 years after their diagnosis of prostate cancer,[5] which makes it a highly manageable condition for most men. In fact, prostate cancer is so manageable for the majority of men that the problem comes in how best to diagnose or treat those patients with no symptoms. Many patients with early prostate cancer will have no signs at all, but they will be diagnosed via an incidental finding of a raised PSA if they request the test. But is having a PSA test enough to make a diagnosis of cancer, and could we be doing more harm than good by potentially investigating or treating men for a condition that might not display any symptoms for the next 20 years? This is the biggest problem we face in trying to tackle screening and the appropriate treatment for prostate cancer.

Myth buster: true or false?

Myth: a family history of breast or ovarian cancer could increase my chance of prostate cancer.

True. Inherited mutations of the BRCA1 or BRCA2 genes, which are usually associated with an increased risk of breast and ovarian cancer in women, can also increase the risk of prostate cancer in male family members affected by the gene mutation (especially mutations in BRCA2).

Screening for prostate cancer

By far the most common question I am asked when discussing prostate cancer with patients is: 'Should I have a PSA test?' There is currently no national screening programme for prostate cancer. As a result, we rely on a combination of symptoms, blood tests and physical examination to see if someone should be referred to a urologist for further investigations. The prostate specific antigen (PSA) used via a test in diagnosing prostate disease is a protein produced by normal cells in the prostate and also by prostate-cancer cells. We all produce a small amount of PSA, and as we get older and the prostate enlarges, so does the amount of PSA produced. The problem comes because PSA levels rise with age not just in prostatitis and prostate cancer. More worryingly, in highly aggressive cancers, the PSA might be completely unaffected, or might even decrease as the prostate gland is obliterated by cancerous tissue.

It might seem, therefore, that PSA testing for prostate cancer is pretty useless because it cannot differentiate between prostate cancer and other forms of benign prostate disease, and it might also miss diagnosing aggressive prostate cancers altogether. But PSA testing does have its uses when applied and interpreted appropriately. My advice is not to get a PSA test without speaking to a health professional first. When assessing prostate disease, it is important to be aware of any symptoms and family history as well as the overall health status of a patient prior to performing the test. These factors might influence a PSA result and could potentially alter how the test is interpreted. I have lost count of the number of patients I have seen with a PSA above normal range who are in their seventies, eighties or nineties, but because the reference ranges for PSA testing are based on a younger demographic, these men are then sent for further investigation, even though they have never needed it but were simply not assessed properly prior to the test.

The other way that PSA testing can be beneficial to prostate health is because repeated tests provide objective and cumulative data. By having serial PSAs taken regularly, it enables us to act on changes in PSA levels early and potentially catch a prostate cancer sooner. A once a year PSA test performed as part of a male MOT would, over several years, provide a helpful trend in PSA levels and would potentially allow a doctor to be able to act on subtle changes earlier on in prostate disease.

Finally, and perhaps most importantly, the PSA test is all we have. When trying to find or investigate men that might have prostate cancer, the PSA test is still an intrinsic part of this process, and we have to use every available tool we can to diagnose and treat patients effectively.

Should I get a PSA test?

Evidence suggests that by screening for prostate cancer with PSA testing, we can reduce prostate cancer deaths by 21 per cent, and the general consensus among prostate cancer charities and organisations is that men should get routinely screened for prostate cancer with a PSA test. Prostate Cancer UK currently advise that all men over 40, irrespective of urinary symptoms, should consider a base-line PSA, which could be used to help predict overall cancer risk. Similarly, the Prostate Cancer Risk Management Programme advises that any men over the age of 50 should speak to their doctor about having a PSA test.

The counter-argument to PSA testing is that by simply having a raised PSA we are likely to over-investigate and potentially do harm to men who turn out not to have cancer. Furthermore, by diagnosing men with prostate cancer too early, we might also end up treating some men who would have died from something else.

If we do more PSA tests, this will inevitably result in more diagnosed cases of prostate cancer, but the test is unable to distinguish between slow-growing tumours that might not need treatment and highly aggressive, fast-growing cancers. A senior urologist whose opinion I greatly value once told me, 'When it comes to prostate cancer, we are great at catching the kittens, but can do little about the tigers.' Overall, a one-off PSA test, taken 'just to check', is very unlikely to be useful. It might falsely reassure an asymptomatic person with aggressive cancer or falsely worry a symptomatic patient who just has a large prostate. But when taken as part of a cumulative data set in conjunction with consulting a doctor, PSA testing can be used effectively to help in the diagnosis and monitoring of prostate cancer.

How can I reduce my chances of getting prostate cancer?

With no national screening programme in place, our goal should be to try to delay the onset and severity of prostate cancer for as long as possible. Although we cannot stop ourselves from getting older, there are various measures that we can take to reduce our overall risk of developing a cancerous prostate gland.

Lifestyle and weight
We know that men in Western countries, such as the UK, are more likely to get prostate cancer than men in east Asian countries such as China and Japan. When these same Asian men move to a Western environment, their risk of prostate cancer goes up. It is very likely that our diets, which contain less fruit, vegetables and fish, and more meat, dairy, sugar, fat and processed foods, are major contributors to our increased risk of developing prostate cancer.

In addition, the latest research suggests that being overweight or obese is associated with a higher incidence of aggressive or advanced prostate disease. A balanced diet and regular exercise can help you to stay a healthy weight and it will also reduce your cancer risk.

Exercise
Studies looking at the relationship between exercise and prostate cancer have mostly shown that men who exercise

have a reduced risk of the disease. We know that exercise has many other health benefits, and it is likely that it is not exercise alone that reduces the risk of prostate cancer but that people who exercise *also* tend to lead a healthier lifestyle in general, eat better and take better care of their overall health. (See also Chapter 2 for more discussion about diet and exercise.)

Vitamin D

In the last few years there has been considerable interest in the link between vitamin D and general health, and it seems that there is some link between vitamin D supplementation and a reduced risk of prostate cancer.[6] The degree to which supplementation reduces the risk of prostate disease requires further research, but as vitamin D is known to be beneficial in a range of other physiological processes, including positive effects on bones, muscles and some hormones, it might be one area where our overall health might benefit from additional vitamin D supplementation. It is, however, worth noting that excess vitamin D supplementation can result in toxicity and cause kidney and bone problems. If you think you might be suffering with low levels of vitamin D, you should consult your doctor.

Dairy and calcium

As an adult, we need about 700mg of calcium each day. This is relatively easy to achieve, as one standard-sized cup of milk provides about 300mg. Current evidence suggests that there is a small increase in the risk of developing prostate cancer in people who have very high intakes of dietary calcium, but excluding dairy or calcium from our diets does not reduce our risk of prostate cancer. As the UK guidance states that a calcium intake up to 1,500mg per day is safe, the detrimental effects of calcium on our health and prostate would not tend to be seen in levels below this. In practice, this would mean having to drink more than five cups of milk per day, eating more than eight tins of salmon, or just over 200g of cheddar cheese (about half a standard block), to reach unhealthy levels.

Cholesterol

Although prostate cancer has been detected in higher numbers of men with raised cholesterol, it's hard to establish which came first, the cholesterol or the cancer. This is because for most men we do not collect their cholesterol or prostate data early on in their life, and men commonly only start to think about MOTs, prostate and cardiovascular health when they reach middle age. There is some evidence that men with raised cholesterol are at greater risk of developing high-grade prostate cancer (the rapidly growing type), but not at an increased overall risk of prostate disease.

Tomatoes

Tomatoes and tomato-based foods contain lycopene, which is a plant-derived nutrient alleged to have a variety of health benefits. In general, eating lycopene might reduce the risk of developing prostate cancer, but it would not alter the growth of existing disease. Most importantly, whereas having lycopene as part of healthy diet is good (and in particular there is more lycopene in cooked tomatoes than fresh), there is no evidence to suggest that taking lycopene supplements will improve prostate health.

Vitamins or supplements that probably don't work
There is a variety of other vitamins and supplements that claim to reduce our chances of developing prostate cancer. These include soya, selenium, vitamin E, multivitamins, pomegranate, flaxseed and turmeric. But there is no good evidence to suggest that any of these foods or vitamins are beneficial for prostate health, and in terms of prostate cancer specifically, some (such as vitamin E) might even increase our cancer risk.[7]

We can't always blame the prostate

Although prostate disease is fundamentally linked to urinary flow, it is important to stress that difficulty passing urine normally is not automatically linked to a defective prostate gland. Whenever I see patients with urinary symptoms, one of the simplest things we can do is look at lifestyle and, in particular, what we eat and drink. Simple steps you can take to improve your own urinary flow include:

- Reducing or avoiding caffeinated drinks such as tea, coffee and cola; drinking a lot of fluids in general, especially later in the day; and spicy foods.
- Make sure you are not constipated.
- Look at medications that you might be taking, including decongestants, antihistamines, antidepressants or water-tablets (diuretics).

- I usually refer patients who have urinary symptoms to urology specialists once we have excluded pros- tate disease and lifestyle issues or infection. The specialist can then look in detail at urinary flow and function.

Prostate in a walnut-shell

Our understanding of prostate disease has progressed tremendously in the last few decades. Treatment for non- cancerous and cancerous conditions have improved, and patients are now able to live fuller, longer lives without being burdened by the effects of a dysfunctional urinary system. The general consensus is that if we live long enough, most of us will suffer with either a large or a cancerous prostate, or both, but this does not necessarily translate to the death sentence or lifelong catheter use that was once the inevitable outcome of prostate disease. When it comes to BPH, surgery is becoming less invasive and more successful than ever before, and newer treatments for prostate cancer mean that record numbers of men are surviving decades after their initial diagnosis.

The issue for prostate disease really comes in the form of screening. For many men it feels that prostate cancer screen- ing is still ambiguous, conflicting and largely ineffective. At present, the best we can do is look towards reducing our chances of getting prostate cancer, rather than relying on a screening programme that might diagnose us too early or be ineffective in catching the cancers that we really needed to treat. Prevention is always better than cure, and until we have a definitive screening programme in place, we have to make an individual judgement about how we manage risk and what measures we are prepared to take to maximise our own health.

Summary

- Our urinary flow is intrinsically linked to our prostate gland. As we get older, testosterone makes it grow, and this can reduce our ability to urinate easily.
- There are a range of problems that can affect the prostate, from inflammation and infection, to slow benign enlargement, to cancer.
- Prostate cancer is the most common cancer in men, accounting for a quarter of all cancer diagnoses.
- PSA tests are vital for monitoring prostate disease, but they cannot by themselves be reliably used to diagnose prostate cancer.
- There remains no national screening programme for prostate cancer.
- You can reduce your risk of developing prostate cancer by:

  1 Avoiding being overweight
  2 Taking regular exercise
  3 Avoiding excessive amounts of calcium
  4 Eating a healthy, balanced diet including plenty of tomatoes
  5 Considering supplementing with vitamin D
  6 Getting a regular health MOT looking at overall prostate health and a PSA test

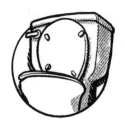

CASE STUDY

When you really need to pee

As a junior doctor in urology, one of the primary skills one is expected to master is the insertion of a male catheter. Catheters are basically long plastic tubes introduced directly up through the penis and into the bladder. For most of us, the concept of having a catheter fitted is eye-watering, but some of the worst pain I have ever seen in men is from those patients who are desperate to urinate but due to an enlarged prostate they are unable to do so. Imagine needing the toilet and not being able to go, but not just holding on for a few minutes, but being unable to pass anything hour after hour, the pain and urge to urinate continuing to build up and being helpless to do anything about it. For those men, having a catheter inserted can make an astonishing difference, and the initial discomfort of having the catheter fitted is easily worth the relief that comes with the ability to pass urine again. Learning to successfully insert a catheter is a combination of theory and practice, and despite understanding the anatomy there is no substitute for practically trying to insert a 40cm floppy plastic tube up through a man's penis while he is writhing in agony.

My first ever practical procedure as a junior doctor was assisting my urological registrar to insert a catheter for a 68-year-old gentleman, Lloyd, who had come in with urinary retention resulting from a large prostate gland. Lloyd had not passed any urine for the last nine hours, and despite sitting in a warm bath, trying to relax and even drinking a coffee (this was not medically advised), he had not passed more than a few drops since the night before. By the time we saw him, Lloyd was in obvious agony, and as this was my first surgical job, I was keen to impress and asked if I could place the catheter, not knowing how difficult it would prove to be. After helping me set up the equipment and gain consent, my registrar sat back in the relative's chair next to the patient and allowed me to attempt the procedure.

After cleaning the area and inserting two large tubes of numbing gel into the man's urethra, I started to feed the catheter into his penis and guide it along until it hit the obstruction, which I presumed was his prostate. Obviously, one cannot simply ram the catheter in harder to get past a blockage, as this can cause severe trauma to the urethra, prostate and surrounding structures, but despite every effort, I could not get the catheter to pass any further. Indeed, I could feel the tube buckling and twisting in the shaft of his penis as I tried to thread it along with increased frustration. After about five minutes, I had gained little progress, and poor Lloyd's pain appeared to be increasing. After looking to my registrar for help, she suggested a few manoeuvres and techniques that might allow me to pass the catheter and also suggested that we actually try a wider diameter tube that could have more success in maintaining its course and direction. Already sympathising with the agonising pain this poor man was going through, I felt under enormous pressure to get this bigger tube in without causing more pain or distress. But just as before, once I hit the prostate I was unable to pass the catheter any further.

Taking the advice of my senior, I pushed with a little more force, and I watched as Lloyd sat bolt upright, and proceeded to vomit all over me. At this point I released the catheter and, just about maintaining my composure, asked if I could go to change, all the while wiping off bits of carrot from my plastic apron. I was hoping that as I obtained a fresh gown and tried to shed the stench of vomit from my person that when I returned the catheter would have been inserted for me, as obviously I was not going to accomplish this task on my own. To my horror, when I got back to the cubicle Lloyd had a fresh gown on and a fresh catheter pack was sitting next to him, my registrar eagerly waiting for me to attempt yet again, a broad grin on her face. This time, and with her help, however, I successfully managed to pass the catheter further than before, but before hitting the bladder, a moderate amount of blood appeared in the catheter tube.

'Don't worry,' my registrar said. 'This will be due to the local trauma of you pushing on the poor guy's prostate so much. Keep going, it'll be fine.'

Nervous about doing more harm, I proceeded to thread the catheter forward at such a slow rate it must have been moving at around a centimetre every few minutes. All the while Lloyd was still rolling around the bed begging for me to just hurry up. It was around this point that seeing the blood in the catheter, combined with the stench of old vomit on my person, and the fact that it was a boiling August afternoon, I started to notice how hot I felt. In fact, the more I thought about it, the more I realised I was sweating a lot.

'Wow, it's really hot in here,' I said to my registrar, trying to keep things jovial and light, but really this was my way of indicating that something in my own body was going horribly wrong.

'Just keep going,' she said, completely avoiding looking at me and studying the notes. 'You're almost there.'

But by now I was feeling very hot indeed, and I had also noticed that my vision had started to get rather hazy at the edges.

'One last push!' she said to me, looking at the catheter, as I then finally hit the bladder and a gush of yellow fluid shot down the tube and started to immediately fill the catheter bag on the side of the bed. Lloyd let out a cry of relief.

With the procedure successful, and crystal-clear urine now flowing joyously through the tube, I proceeded to smoothly and stylishly sink to the floor. To my registrar it must have looked as if I had suddenly accessed an invisible elevator and had pressed the button for ground. Although remaining conscious, I remember sitting up on the tiled floor of the cubicle, my head resting on the rapidly filling bag containing Lloyd's urine. Although my vision had almost completely disappeared at this point, I remember knowing where I was because I could feel the heat of Lloyd's warm urine in the catheter bag that was now propping up my left cheek.

During handover at the end of the day, my registrar told me that she had never laughed so hard during an on-call and she was greatly looking forward to working with me again. Lloyd also appeared to be happier, now suffering no discomfort, and having drained just less than a litre of urine. Finally, I was also feeling better, having changed into scrubs, but reluctant to collect the carrier bag in my locker which now contained my shirt and trousers saturated in my sweat and a combination of someone else's vomit and urine. On my way to the car, I binned the clothes, and recall thinking that medicine was not turning out to be as glamorous as I had imagined it would be.

CHAPTER 9

What to Do Next

You have decided to take a more proactive approach to your health, so what should you do next? There are a near infinite number of companies offering different ways to improve your well-being, and deciding on which products to buy, or which strategies to adopt, can be a daunting task. We live in a society where expectations of how we should look and behave are hard to reconcile with what most of us can actually achieve. We work longer hours than we should, exercise for many people is a painful and unrewarding process, and try as hard as we might, many of us cannot rid ourselves of our inner anxieties and disruptive thoughts. Some of us might even suffer with medical conditions that rob us of the chance to live a life we dreamt of. This can make us feel cheated or resentful and look to blame others for shortcomings that are out of our control.

Therefore, once we have made the decision to take better care of ourselves, perhaps the biggest hurdle we face is not which supplement to take, which gym to join or which blood test to have, but how we go about taking responsibility for the changes that we need to make, and what practical steps are needed to achieve the outcomes we want. This chapter provides the six steps required to start your journey towards better health.

Select a realistic goal

It might seem obvious, but simply wanting to 'be healthier' or 'improve my wellness' are nebulous concepts that can be particularly daunting and provide no practical reference or focus on what you actually need to do. Therefore, the most important initial step is to decide what aspect of your health you want to address. This might take the form of a specific lifestyle goal such as getting fit or losing weight, it might be to get a regular health check, or it might even be to look into resolving some niggling health issues that you have put to the back of your mind.

It is not essential to know in what form the journey will take, but by knowing what you want to achieve in terms of your health and wellness it gives you something to aim for. If you feel that you are generally quite healthy, eat well, exercise and live a healthy lifestyle, perhaps getting a health check is a suitable starting point, as many health problems such as high cholesterol or high blood pressure are generally asymptomatic, and other symptoms such as low testosterone might just be confused with the pace of day-to-day life.

Make time for your mental well-being

When patients attend my clinic wishing to improve or change their lifestyle, this is usually motivated by a desire to improve their physical health. Most men subsequently devote many hours a week to introducing exercise regimes, preparing meals or monitoring their physical observations such as blood pressure or number of steps walked per day. But whereas we see this physical change as a logical step towards better health, we rarely spend the same amount of time or effort on our mental well-being.

Technology has connected us with the world and other people in a way that we never would have imagined a few years ago. But whereas this might have its advantages, it can make it very hard to be able to switch off or say no. Our jobs and lifestyles mean that we can be contacted at any time, and we no longer leave work behind us at the office. In addition, social media provides a constant intrusive and distorted image of what the world is like. Therefore, if you are serious about improving your overall health, in addition to the physical steps that you take it is essential to try to assign yourself at least 30 minutes a day where you do not answer text messages or emails and give yourself that much-needed time in which to reflect.

Having time to self-reflect, ruminate and think over

things in our minds is a crucial aspect of maintaining our mental wellness. Many cases of mental illness are made worse by external pressures that make us feel overloaded or pressured, but having even that brief time to ourselves can help us to rationalise worries and concerns, set priorities and put plans in place.

When it comes to which psychological programme or technique is the most beneficial, there are many to choose from and, much like diets, every few years another new one is produced. But in practice it is really just about finding something that fits your life and personality. I certainly would not advocate that everyone needs to start going to therapy, and many men are able to use their exercise time as a way to give them that space to think and reflect. Even just going for a walk can be enough to allow us to disconnect from the pressures of the world and help us to prepare for the next challenge ahead.

Remember what you were made for

It has taken us millions of years to evolve into the creatures we are today, but over the last century the way we function and live our lives has been radically at odds with what we were engineered to do. Most of us spend our days sitting at work, we have easy access to high-calorie foods and very few of us need to worry about the threat of attack from wild animals.

Although progress in industry and technology has allowed us to live more sedentary and comfortable lives, our bodies have not caught up with this change in social behaviour. Put bluntly, we are simply not built to spend all day looking at screens and eating doughnuts. As a child, I used to think it very odd that my friend's hamster would suddenly get up out of its bed and run on a wheel that went nowhere; however, looking at the recent surge in popularity of fitness centres and gyms, in particular the use of treadmills, the irony is not lost. Our lives are now generally so devoid of movement that we have to think of novel and interesting ways to provide that physical stimulus that genetically our bodies and minds crave.

If you are in a job that has little or no physical element to it, finding an activity that burns calories and gets your body moving is essential. A walk in the evenings three times a week does not count. The key is to find something that is challenging, makes you tired and out of breath but is ultimately enjoyable and repeatable. Deep down, we are still cavemen and our bodies will thank us if we fight the occasional tiger.

Be patient

When it comes to improving our health and well-being, it is important to stress that this process is a marathon and not a sprint. Although it is possible to see some positive changes in our bodies, both physically and mentally, in only a few weeks after starting a new programme these changes tend to be small and superficial. Our bodies are very good at resisting change; therefore, it can take many months for us to see the true potential of any lifestyle measures we undertake now. We see ourselves in the mirror every day, which can make it hard to step back and objectively appreciate the positive changes we have made.

Unless you have a specific short-term goal, such as trying to lose weight for a holiday, you must be prepared to be patient. Beware of shortcuts, and as tempting as products with slogans such as 'get your dream body in six weeks' might be, they should be avoided. This is not because they don't work, but because they tend to result in a yo-yo effect. Many food-restricting diets are able to achieve good results within a relatively short period of time because they reduce the total amount of calories consumed. But the diets themselves are either unhealthy or monotonous. Either way, they are unsustainable, and when a client finishes the course, they go back to whatever bad eating and lifestyle habits they had before. Unsurprisingly, the weight also comes back, too. Any diet we undertake should not really be a diet at all. Instead, we should aim for moderate and incremental changes in the way we eat as part of a wider improvement in our overall lifestyle – we should build good habits. Simply advising people to eat less and have more fruit and vegetables is not sexy, however, and it does not sell books or apps.

How old are you?

What we perceive as 'normal for age' depends on our interactions with friends and family, as well as how we are influenced by society and culture. This means that it is easy for us to fall into the narrative that being overweight, tired and grumpy is normal for a middle-aged man. But, as discussed in Chapter 1 on testosterone deficiency, sometimes society can falsely reaffirm our belief that our symptoms are normal simply because we have reached a certain milestone.

My advice is to look at how you feel about yourself. Irrespective of your age, look at your quality of life and critically assess whether there are aspects that you are unhappy with. Ask yourself questions like:

- Do I have the energy I want?
- Am I going to the toilet too often?
- Am I struggling to make gains in the gym or feel that I am getting fatter?
- Are my erections less strong than they used to be?

If the answer to any of these questions is yes, or you feel that there is any aspect of your health or well-being that is affecting you negatively, do not simply accept this as normal. Speak to your doctor, get a high-quality and personalised health check, change your lifestyle in a positive way, or if you are not sure what to do, a good starting point might be to get the health check offered by the NHS.

Get a health check

We can all start to make positive changes to our lifestyle by getting a health check. Health checks are particularly useful for several reasons:

1. They provide us with objective data about the current state of our health.

2. They can give us information about our potential risk of future disease (such as high cholesterol or diabetes).

3. They can help us explain why we might be suffering with symptoms due to a condition that we did not know about (such as low testosterone).

4. They can also be used to help motivate us and work as a guide towards an overall change in health behaviour.

From the age of 40, the NHS offers a health check to everyone who has not already been diagnosed with significant underlying cardiovascular disease and some other medical problems such as diabetes or kidney disease. It specifically looks for diabetes, kidney, stroke and heart disease, and its introduction in 2009 saw a major shift in the way the NHS approaches healthcare. But is 40 too late to think about health checks, and should we be screening for more than just cardiovascular risk?

We know that damage to our arteries from conditions such as high cholesterol actually begins in our twenties. We also know that the diets of younger men tend to be less healthy than later in life when disposable income, education and access to better quality food is more available. Add the fact that testosterone levels tend to decline after the age of 30, and over 2.1 million people in the UK have a diagnosis of high blood pressure under the age of 45. Realistically, by the time you are in your mid-forties, it is likely that you have had several decades of potential cardiovascular damage. But would offering health checks before the age of 30 provide better long-term outcomes for patients? The argument against providing health checks for the young is that testing all men at the age of 20 for heart disease is not only likely to yield a poor pick-up rate, but also, owing to the perception of invincible youth, it is unlikely to generate much interest. What, then, is the best age to get a health check?

In reality, there is no single age that is best to get a health check, but a one-off screening is unlikely to provide the data you need for a lifetime of health, irrespective of what age it is performed. The aim of a health check should be to find out what your base level of health is, and then to repeat your screening at specific intervals to assess the progress you make and overall improvements in health. But even if you decide to get a health check, with such a large range of products available, it can be hard to know which one is best. Private health-check services range in price from a few hundred pounds to several thousand pounds. Tests can include a range of practical assessments such as fitness levels, body fat measurement and memory tests, as well as different forms of imaging such as X-rays, heart traces or even MRI scans. This can make it even harder to decide what actually defines a quality health check, as bigger is not necessarily better.

In summary, when looking for a health check, the best way to decide if it is right for you is to see if the service addresses your individual health needs, concerns and risk factors. Are you really being listened to or is this just a tick-box exercise with pre-defined tests and pre-determined outcomes? The best health checks are those that look at you as a person; they do not need to cost the earth, but getting the right test done at the right time can make a crucial difference in how you approach your health and well-being. In the chart overleaf you will find some tips on what to be aware of when considering a health check.

A final note

Part of the reason why so many of us fail to achieve our goals in improving our health is a lack of true self-belief, reaffirmed by the social construct that taunts us as we get older. This is not to say that we might not be happy, but many of us end up falling into the narrative of being tired, overweight and emotionally blunted middle-aged men, existing from one day to the next without really living up to, or maximising, who we could be.

This does not have to be the case, however. I am not suggesting that we should all quit our jobs and travel the world, or live every day as if it's our last. The aim of this book is to educate men on the different aspects of their health so that they can better understand their own bodies and make improved health choices, as well as empowering them to break away from what is the accepted normal. You can just get older, fatter, more tired and lonelier, but you don't have to. Whether it is treating baldness, getting fitter or tackling male-hormone deficiency, we can all make individual changes at various levels that allow us to live better and longer lives. Statistics state that as men we are doomed from the start, but I propose that we do not have to accept who we are just because genetics, work or society tells us that is who we should be.

What to look for in a health check

Health check service	What it offers	What it means
The number of health measurements or blood tests provided	Some health checks boast statements such as 'We perform over 100 different blood tests with every health check.'	The total number of health parameters measured in a health check is often a deliberately misleading number that might include tests irrelevant to you. A quality health check will tailor the investigations carried out to match your individual concerns and risk factors.
The structure of the assessment	Many health checks suggest a pre-screening questionnaire, a fixed set of questions with yes/no answers, and a number of pre-determined blood tests or scans than are done in advance.	A 65-year-old man with prostate disease does not require the same health check as a 30-year-old diabetic. Your assessment should include open questions about your current state of health and risk factors, and address any symptoms, worries or concerns you have. It should not just be a tick-box exercise.

How much it costs	Some health checks can cost thousands of pounds and include MRI scans of the brain, liver ultrasounds, bone density measurements and many other specialist tests.	There is an illusion in medicine that testing for more things is always better. In fact, in health checks, specialist scans are often unnecessary for the majority of people. Although some complex investigations might be useful, they should only be performed in the context of a specific issue or problem identified during the screening consultation, not as a matter of routine.
What do you do with the results?	Many health checks include your results in a summary booklet or guide. Some even try to make it easier to understand by offering a 'green is okay, red you're in trouble' traffic-light system. Ultimately, however, the advice is to go back to your own doctor to action anything that is flagged up as abnormal.	It is the responsibility of the provider offering the health check to discuss your results with you. In addition, any health check should result in a plan of action that addresses all problems identified. The only time a referral to another clinician should occur is if a specific medical issue is highlighted that requires specialist input.

CHAPTER 10

What is a Doctor Worth?

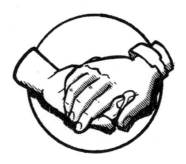

When the health service fails in some aspect of care, either as waiting times, missed diagnoses or ease of access to a doctor, general practitioners are the usual target for media and political blame. This is not because the job of a GP is any less pressured or differs in workload from any other medical speciality. It is because the concept of what a GP does is understandable, and most patients have a reasonable idea about how they hope their patient journey will progress when they come to see their doctor. Because the concept of what general practice means is so straightforward, it makes it an easy target when things go wrong. We're all familiar with newspaper articles with titles such as 'GP missed my diagnosis of cancer' or 'I had to wait four weeks for my appointment and now it's too late'. It is this combination of media bashing and politically driven targeting of general practice that makes overall satisfaction of being a GP rated at an all-time low.

When I mentioned the reasons for the high amount of burnout in GPs to my friend who works as a doctor in intensive care, he was completely unaware of this problem, and had never experienced any of this animosity towards his speciality. The reason for this goes back to our perceived understanding of what the job entails. Although we can all understand how family medicine works, no one can say the same for intensive-care doctors, as very few people know what they actually do. More than 90 per cent of clinical contacts with doctors are with a GP, which means that it is essential that we have a broad understanding of all medical, psychological and social aspects of care; however, the problem here is that it also means we cannot be specialists in everything. I once had a new patient who questioned my knowledge as a doctor because I had to google his medical condition, which I was not familiar with. It turned out that his glycogen storage disorder had a prevalence of less than one in a million, but my lack of knowledge immediately marked me out as inferior in his eyes.

With this constant demoralisation of GPs, there has been a slow decline in recruitment towards the speciality. I recently had medical students who sat in with me during my clinics and who both openly said that they had no interest in pursuing a career in general practice as they hated the way that they would be portrayed in the media and were put off by the abuse we regularly received from irate or disrespectful patients.

With that in mind, it might be easy to become despondent or lose interest in a speciality, which, when given the chance, can be the most rewarding of all medical disciplines. This is because as GPs we look after patients holistically. We are not sub-specialists dealing with only one part of the body or looking after rare glycogen storage disorders. We are responsible for every aspect of a patient's care: from medical, to psychological and social. We get to know people from their birth, we follow them through childhood, and we support them as they grow old. Many times, we are also there when they die. It is this link that GPs build with families, often over many years, that can be so important as someone reaches the end of their life. When patients or families might be anxious, angry or scared, this is often a time that as a GP we can really do our most to help.

I had known Gerald since I joined the practice, initially as a registrar, over 12 years ago. He had just become a grandfather and my first introduction to him was actually for a consultation for his grandson whom he had brought in with a cough. Gerald was in his early seventies and was the type of grandfather most children would want to have. He was energetic and full of life, he appeared to be younger than his years, and he constantly irritated his son and daughter-in-law by behaving in a juvenile fashion around his grandson, much to his grandson's delight. Grandpa Gerald was well liked by the whole family, and he looked after his grandson four days a week while the parents were at work.

Gerald had been widowed 30 years ago; he had

never remarried and so he spent most of his time alone. Consequently, the introduction of a grandson had given him a new purpose in life, and one that he did not take for granted. Therefore, over the next few years, whenever Gerald's grandson was ill and needed to see a doctor, it was him that brought the child to see me. On reflection, I think I only ever met the parents of the child once or twice.

After a few years of getting to know him, Gerald attended because he had had problems passing urine and, although he was used to getting up in the night, it had become so bothersome that he decided he needed to do something about it. Gerald said that there were some days where he was getting up four or five times a night just to go to the toilet and, in addition to his poor sleep, Gerald had also felt more fatigued recently, his urinary flow had really diminished and he thought he might have noticed some blood in his urine on a few occasions, although he could not be sure.

Gerald had a few blood tests and a physical examination, which was essentially normal, but his PSA (explained on page 221) had come back very high. As a result, Gerald was referred to the urologists, where he underwent further tests, scans and a biopsy, and was eventually told that he had prostate cancer. The good news was that the cancer was still localised to the prostate gland and had not spread. As a consequence, the agreement with the urologist was to watch and wait, there was no urgency for treatment and he could have medical therapy to reduce the size and impact of his prostate and make him urinate better.

Over the next few months, Gerald's symptoms improved, and he started to look more like his old self. His energy came back, and I saw less and less of him in clinic. Gradually, Gerald's visits to the GP returned to a similar pattern as they were before his diagnosis, and I tended only to see him when he brought in his grandson. Amazingly, even five years on, Gerald remained largely unaffected by his prostate cancer, which he referred to as an annoyance although entirely manageable. He did not particularly enjoy the side effects of the injections that treated his cancer, which reduced his testosterone to near zero levels. He said that while he did not care about the lack of sex drive or erections, as that wasn't really a concern any more, he did find the night sweats and hot flushes quite uncomfortable, and he also felt less motivated in life than he used to. But, overall, the benefits outweighed the negatives.

Then, Gerald had a particularly bad chest infection, and during a brief stay in hospital, he was diagnosed with leukaemia. Gerald had attributed many of the symptoms of his leukaemia to his prostate cancer treatment, as both can cause fatigue, night sweats and weight loss. The two cancers were unrelated, according to the haematologist – Gerald had just been very unlucky.

Whether it was due to his age, as Gerald was now in his eighties, or the fact that he was already fighting another cancer, Gerald's health appeared to decline quite rapidly after his diagnosis. He underwent a few courses of chemotherapy, but this was complicated by several episodes of sepsis, for which he was admitted to hospital, as well as anaemia, which meant that he needed multiple blood transfusions. Within one year of diagnosis, Gerald had deteriorated so much that he was transferred to the palliative care team and put forward for supportive treatment and care while all active cancer therapy was stopped. Rather than being able to see me, I ended up visiting Gerald in his own home several times over the next few months, and with increased frequency. Gerald's son, daughter-in-law, grandson (now aged 12), as well as his granddaughter, were almost always there, too.

Gerald seemed quite stoical about this situation and never really complained about his illness, but I think that his family had a hard time dealing with his decline in health. Gerald's son was more unemotional than I remembered him, he often appeared detached and would always avoid difficult or uncomfortable discussions about his father's health. One morning, I was asked if I could attend a home visit to see Gerald as his son was worried that he appeared difficult to rouse and was unable to communicate.

When I arrived at the house, Gerald's grandchildren were at school but his son and daughter-in-law were there, and obviously anxious. I went to assess Gerald, and he was indeed very flat. His breathing rate was around one breath every five to ten seconds, and he appeared unresponsive to all my efforts to wake him.

'How long has he been like this?' I asked.

'Probably the last 24 hours I guess,' his daughter-in-law replied, 'but he is much worse this morning.'

I looked back at Gerald, and then up to his family who were waiting expectantly for my miracle answer. I remember saying clearly to them, 'I think he's dying. You might want to come and just sit with him for now. He may know you're here, and I'm sure it would mean a lot. I can go in the other room.'

'How long has he got?' his son asked. 'Is there nothing else you can do? I'm not ready for this.'

'I'm really sorry,' I replied. 'I can't say for sure, but I think it's soon, his breathing is really shallow and I just think you should be ready.'

At this, I was quite surprised to see Gerald's son fling his arms into the air and shout, 'I can't do this now!' He then stormed out of the room, his wife following just behind, calling his name in an effort to convince him to come back.

This was one of the most awkward moments in my medical career. I was now left alone with a man I did not know particularly well, who might die in front of me. I wanted to run out and try to convince Gerald's son to come back and be with his father in his last moments, but I also felt that I could not risk leaving someone who could be about to take his final breath. Rationally, I knew that he probably wasn't conscious, but I just felt unable to live with the idea that the man in front of me might be scared, and no one should have to die alone. I pulled up the chair and sat next to him. I think I recall talking out loud, making inane small talk to try to distract myself from how uncomfortable I felt.

At this point, Gerald started to elongate the pauses in between his breaths. This would then be interspersed with sudden episodes of rapid breathing, known as Cheyne-Stokes breathing, and is often seen in the final moments of life.

'I really think you need to come in now!' I shouted to the family who remained somewhere off in the back of the house, but I heard nothing. 'It's really important!' But still no one materialised.

There are certain types of doctors who are happy with being touchy-feely. They often put a hand on a patient's arm if giving bad news, or may prefer to shake hands at the start of every consultation, or they might even offer a hug in difficult situations. I am definitely not one of those doctors. In fact, I have always separated myself from unnecessarily touching my patients, as it would not fit with my personality. But this felt beyond normal. Not knowing what else to do, I reflexively reached out and held Gerald's hand, giving it a gentle squeeze, just in case he knew that I was there. A few seconds later, Gerald took one more deep breath and then exhaled for the last time.

I didn't really know what to do next, so I just sat and waited for a few minutes. Perhaps unrealistically waiting for him to start breathing again, or open his eyes, or sit up, but probably more because I felt Gerald deserved a moment's dignity.

His son came back in a while later, and I informed him that his father had passed. Within moments, his daughter-in-law was on the phone to their family, breaking the news. Simultaneously, Gerald's son proceeded to go over to his father, stared at him for a moment, and then turned to me, shook my hand, and thanked me for being there when his dad needed him – I was not sure if he meant just now or over the years. I had a brief conversation with them both about bereavement services, and after making sure to stress how important it was that they took care of each other during this difficult time, I went back to my car and started my afternoon clinic 15 minutes later, as if it was just another ordinary day.

Many people might think that they understand general practice. But we do more than just hand out pills and order tests. Our job is to be the patient's advocate. No matter the cause, as GPs we support our patients through their journey, whether it is via medication, providing the link with hospital specialities, being someone they can talk to or just by being there for them when no one else will.

References

Chapter 1

1 Tajar, A., Forti, G., O'Neill, T., et al., 'Characteristics of secondary, primary, and compensated hypogonadism in aging men: Evidence from the European Male Ageing Study', *Journal of Clinical Endocrinology Metabolism*, 2010; 95(4): 1810–18; Wu, F., Tajar, A., Beynon, J., et al., 'Identification of late-onset hypogonadism in middle-aged and elderly men', *New England Journal of Medicine*, 2010; 363(2): 123–35

2 Bain. J., 'The many faces of testosterone', *Clinical Interventions in Aging*, 2007; 2(4): 567–76

3 Hackett, G., Kirby, M., Edwards, D., et al., 'British Society for Sexual Medicine Guidelines on Adult Testosterone Deficiency, with statements for UK Practice', *Journal of Sexual Medicine*, 2017; 14(12): 1504–23

4 'ISSM Quick reference guide on testosterone deficiency for men', International Society for Sexual Medicine (September 2015) https://professionals.issm.info/wp-content/uploads/sites/2/2018/05/ISSM-Quick-Reference-Guide-on-TD.pdf [Accessed 22 December 2020]

5 Gray, P., 'The descent of a man's testosterone', *Proceedings of the National Academy of Sciences of the United States of America*, 2011; 108(39):16141–2

6 Leproult, R., Van Cauter, E., 'Effect of 1 week of sleep restriction on testosterone levels in young healthy men', *Journal of the American Medical Association*, 2011305(21): 2173–4

7 Jiang, M., Xin, J., Zou, Q., Shen, J. A., 'Research on the relationship between ejaculation and serum testosterone level in men', *Journal of Zejiang University Science*, 2003; 4(2): 236–40

8 Exton, M., Krüger, T., Bursch, N., et al., 'Endocrine response to masturbation-induced orgasm in healthy men following a 3-week sexual abstinence', *World Journal of Urology*, 2001; 19(5): 377–82

9 Bhasin, S., Cunningham, G., Hayes, et al., 'Testosterone therapy in men with androgen deficiency syndromes: An endocrine society clinical practice guideline', *Journal of Clinical Endocrinology & Metabolism*, 2010; 95(6): 2536–59; Dandona, P., Rosenberg, M.T., 'A practical guide to male hypogonadism in the primary care setting', *International Journal of Clinical Practice*, 2010; 64(6): 682–96

10 Ramasamy, R., Fisher, E., Schlegel, P., 'Testosterone replacement and prostate cancer', *Indian Journal of Urology*, 2012; 28(2): 123–8

Chapter 2

1 The top 10 causes of death. World Health Organization December, 2020. https://www.who.int/news-room/fact-sheets/detail/the-top-10-causes-of-death [Accessed December 2020]

2 Li, J. J., Corey, E.J., *Drug Discovery: Practices, Processes, and Perspectives*, Wiley Publishers, 2013

3 Alberti, F., 'John Hunter's Heart', *Annals of the Royal College of Surgeons (Suppl)*, 2013; 95: 168–169

4 Ferry, A., Anand, A., Strachan, F., et al., 'Presenting symptoms in men and women diagnosed with myocardial infarction, using sex-specific criteria', *Journal of the American Heart Association*, 2019; 8(17): e012307

5 Bots, S., Peters, S., Woodward, M., 'Sex differences in coronary heart disease and stroke mortality: A global assessment of the effect of ageing between 1980 and 2010', *British Medical Journal (Global Health)*, 2017; 2(2): e000298

6 Tawakol, A., Ishai, A., Takx, R., et al., 'Relation between resting amygdalar activity and cardiovascular events: a longitudinal and cohort study', *Lancet*, 2017; 389(10071): 834–84

7 Health Survey for England 2017 [NS], (2018) https://digital.nhs.uk/data-and-information/publications/statistical/health-survey-for-england/2017 [Accessed September 2020]

8 Phillips, D., Curtice, J., Phillips, M., Perry J., *British Social Attitudes: The 35th Report*, National Centre for Social Research (2018)

9 'A Government Statistical Service perspective on official estimates of calorie consumption', Office for National Statistics (2016) https://www.ons.gov.uk/peoplepopulationandcommunity/

healthandsocialcare/conditionsanddiseases/methodologies/
agovernmentstatisticalserviceperspectiveonofficialestimatesofcalorie
consumption#summary [Accessed September 2020]

Chapter 3

1 McManus, S., Bebbington, P., Jenkins, R., Brugha, T. (eds), (2016) 'Mental health and well-being in England: Adult Psychiatric Morbidity Survey 2014', Leeds: NHS Digital https://assets.publishing.service.gov. uk/government/uploads/system/uploads/attachment_data/file/556596/ apms-2014-full-rpt.pdf [Accessed October 2020]

2 Simms, C., Scowcroft, E., Isaksen, M., et al., 'Suicide Statistics Report 2019, The Samaritans', https://media.samaritans.org/documents/ SamaritansSuicideStatsReport_2019_Full_report.pdf [Accessed September 2020]

3 Hall, W., Degenhardt, L., 'Cannabis use and the risk of developing a psychotic disorder', *World Psychiatry*, 2008; 7(2): 68–71

4 Gandal, M., Haney, J., Parikshak, N., et al., 'Shared molecular neuropathology across major psychiatric disorders parallels polygenic overlap', *Science*, 2018; 359(6376): 693–7

5 'Depression in adults with a chronic physical health problem: recognition and management', Clinical guideline [CG91] National Institute for Health and Care Excellence (NICE), 2009 https://www.nice.org.uk/guidance/cg91/chapter/ Context#step-1-recognition-assessment-and-initial-management-in-primary-care-and-general-hospital [Accessed September 2020]

6 Moussavi, S., Chatterji, S., Verdes, E., et al., 'Depression, chronic disease and decrements in health: Results from the World Health Surveys', *Lancet*, 2007; 370: 851–8

7 'Suicides in the UK: 2017 registrations: Registered deaths in the UK from suicide analysed by sex, age, area of usual residence of the deceased and suicide method', Office of National Statistics (2018) https://www.ons.gov.uk/ peoplepopulationandcommunity/birthsdeathsandmarriages/deaths/ bulletins/suicidesintheunitedkingdom/2017registrations [Accessed November 2020]

8 Callanan, V., Davis, M., 'Gender and suicide method: Do women avoid facial disfiguration?', *Sex Roles*, 2011; 65:867–79

9 Ibid.

10 Netz, Y., 'Is the comparison between exercise and pharmacologic

treatment of depression in the clinical practice guideline of the American College of Physicians Evidence-Based?' *Frontiers in Pharmacology*, 2017; 8: 257

11 O'Neil, A., Quirk, S.E., Housden, S., et al., 'Relationship between diet and mental health in children and adolescents: A systematic review', *American Journal of Public Health*, 2014; 104(10): 31–42

Chapter 4

1 Feldman, H.A., Goldstein, I., Hatzichristou, D.G., et al., 'Impotence and its medical and psychosocial correlates: Results of the Massachusetts Male Aging Study', *Journal of Urology*, 1994; 151(1): 54–61

2 Johannes, C., Araujo, A., Feldman, H., et al., 'Incidence of erectile dysfunction in men 40 to 69 years old: Longitudinal results from the Massachusetts Male Aging Study', *Journal of Urology*, 2000; 163(2):460–3

Chapter 5

1 Arias-Santiago, S., Arrabal-Polo, M.A., Buendía-Eisman, A., et al., 'Androgenetic alopecia as an early marker of benign prostatic hyperplasia', *Journal of the American Academy of Dermatology*, 2012 66(3): 401–8

2 Polat, E.C., Ozcan, L., Otunctemur, A., Ozbek, E., 'Relation of urinary stone disease with androgenetic alopecia and serum testosterone levels', *Urolithiasis*, 2016; 44(5): 409–13

Chapter 8

1 Krieger, J.N., Lee, S.W., Jeon, J., et al., 'Epidemiology of prostatitis', *International Journal of Antimicrobial Agents*, 2008; 31(1): 85–90

2 'Cancer incidence for common cancers', Cancer Research UK (2017) https://www.cancerresearchuk.org/health-professional/cancer-statistics/incidence/common-cancers-compared#heading-One [Accessed August 2020]

3 Stangelberger, A., Waldert, M., Djavan, B., 'Prostate cancer in elderly men', *Reviews in Urology*, 2008; 10(2): 111–19

4 Bill-Axelson, A., Holmberg, L., Garmo, H., et al., 'Radical prostatectomy or watchful waiting in prostate cancer:

29-year follow-up', *New England Journal of Medicine*, 2018;
13379(24): 2319–29

5 Prostate cancer statistics Cancer Research UK (2017) https://www.
   cancerresearchuk.org/health-professional/cancer-statistics/statistics-by-
   cancer-type/prostate-cancer [Accessed September 2020]

6 'Cancer incidence for common cancers', Cancer Research UK
   (2017) https://www.cancerresearchuk.org/health-professional/
   cancer-statistics/incidence/common-cancers-compared#heading-One
   [Accessed August 2020]

7 Ibid.

Index

Note: page numbers in **bold** refer to diagrams, page numbers in *italics* refer to information contained in tables.